# TIP
of the
# ADHD
# ICEBERG

# TIP of the ADHD ICEBERG

AN ADULT'S GUIDE TO EMBRACING THE HIDDEN LAYERS OF YOUR NEURODIVERGENCE

## DR SAMANTHA HIEW

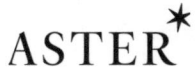

First published in Great Britain in 2025 by Aster, an imprint of
Octopus Publishing Group Ltd
Carmelite House
50 Victoria Embankment
London EC4Y 0DZ
www.octopusbooks.co.uk

An Hachette UK Company
www.hachette.co.uk

The authorized representative in the EEA is Hachette Ireland,
8 Castlecourt Centre, Dublin 15, D15 XTP3, Ireland (email: info@hbgi.ie)

Text copyright © Dr Samantha Hiew 2025
Illustrations credit: Ilana Graham and Mel Four

Distributed in the US by Hachette Book Group
1290 Avenue of the Americas, 4th and 5th Floors
New York, NY 10104

Distributed in Canada by Canadian Manda Group
664 Annette St., Toronto, Ontario, Canada M6S 2C8

All rights reserved. No part of this work may be reproduced or utilized in any form or by any means, electronic or mechanical, including photocopying, recording or by any information storage and retrieval system, without the prior written permission of the publisher.

Dr Samantha Hiew asserts the right to be identified as the author of this work.

ISBN 978-1-78325-646-4
eBook ISBN 978-1-78325-648-8

A CIP catalogue record for this book is available from the British Library.

Typeset in 11.25/14.5 Garamond Premier Pro by Six Red Marbles UK, Thetford, Norfolk

Printed and bound in Great Britain.

1 3 5 7 9 10 8 6 4 2

Commissioning Editor: Louisa Johnson
Project Editor: Rimsha Falak
Copy Editor: Joanna Smith
Creative Director: Mel Four
Production Controller: Sarah Parry

This FSC® label means that materials used for the product have been responsibly sourced.

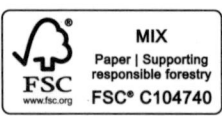

Disclaimer: All reasonable care has been taken in the preparation of this book but the information it contains is not intended to take the place of treatment by a qualified medical practitioner. Before making any changes in your health regime, always consult a doctor. While all the therapies detailed in this book are completely safe if done correctly, you must seek professional advice if you are in any doubt about any medical condition. Any application of the ideas and information contained in this book is at the reader's sole discretion and risk.

**For Raphie and Leo,**
the loves of my life –
I would give you the world if I could.
This book is my offering to your future.

## WHAT PEOPLE THINK ADHD IS

- Fidgety
- Inattentive
- Forgetful
- Tardy
- Hyperactive
- Restless
- Impulsive
- Unmotivated

## WHAT ADHD ACTUALLY INVOLVES

- Impact of early childhood experiences
- Performance feedback sensitivity
- Burnout
- Masking
- Sensory overwhelm
- Different attachment styles
- Overstimulation
- Sleep disorders
- Co-occurring conditions (e.g. autism & anxiety)
- People-pleasing
- Rejection sensitivity dysphoria
- Metabolic differences
- Navigating biases
- Need for community

# Contents

Introduction ... 1

Step 1: Understand It's Not Your Fault ... 13
Step 2: Expect to Discover Co-occurring Conditions ... 41
Step 3: Understand Your Nature ... 77
Step 4: Trace Your Beginnings ... 107
Step 5: Identify Your Emotional Needs ... 143
Step 6: Expect Your Relationships to Change and Adapt ... 177
Step 7: Navigate Your Neurodiversity at Work ... 219
Step 8: Find Your Community ... 249
Step 9: Emerge as Your True Self ... 269

Conclusion: The Journey Ahead ... 301
Glossary ... 303
Source Notes ... 305
Acknowledgements ... 317
Index ... 321

# Introduction

Being diagnosed with attention deficit hyperactivity disorder, or ADHD, later in life can feel like an abrupt awakening – as though your life has been forever changed. Some things may suddenly start to make sense, such as all those times you've been criticized for always being late, or prone to fly off the handle, or you just couldn't seem to apply yourself, much to the dismay of loved ones. To them, it might have seemed as though your life was filled with hedonistic pursuits and destructive tendencies towards yourself and the people around you. Maybe you still sometimes appear a little socially awkward, anxious or depressed, and it can perhaps feel as if you're a mystery to both yourself and others.

However your ADHD makes itself known in your life, it doesn't exist in a vacuum: your upbringing, your culture, your relationships and any other conditions you might have, such as autism, depression or anxiety, all affect your experience as a neurodivergent. Navigating these intersecting areas can be challenging – but it isn't impossible.

This book will guide you through the nuances of neurodiversity, preparing you for the whirlwind that can come after realizing that you are neurodivergent, and also from being recognized as neurodivergent by other people following a diagnosis. Along the way, it will equip you with the essential tools for self-advocacy. I will be drawing on my own lived experience of ADHD and autism as well as my background in medical science to help you process your diagnosis in the context of your whole life – from your personal relationships to the workplace environment. My hope is that you will learn to heal from years of flying under the radar and discover how to prepare yourself for lift-off into the life you want.

## THE ADHD ICEBERG

Having walked this journey myself as a late-diagnosed AuDHDer (somebody who has both ADHD and autistic traits), and having spoken to hundreds of thousands of neurodivergent individuals across eclectic life contexts, cultures and generations, I feel qualified to say I know what you're dealing with if you've recently received a diagnosis.

As part of my work today, I often give talks about neurodiversity, during which one particular graphic has been consistently met with audible gasps and *aha!* moments in the audience. It's the 'female ADHD iceberg' (see below). In it, I've brought together all the other traits that people don't tend to see beyond the surface of the

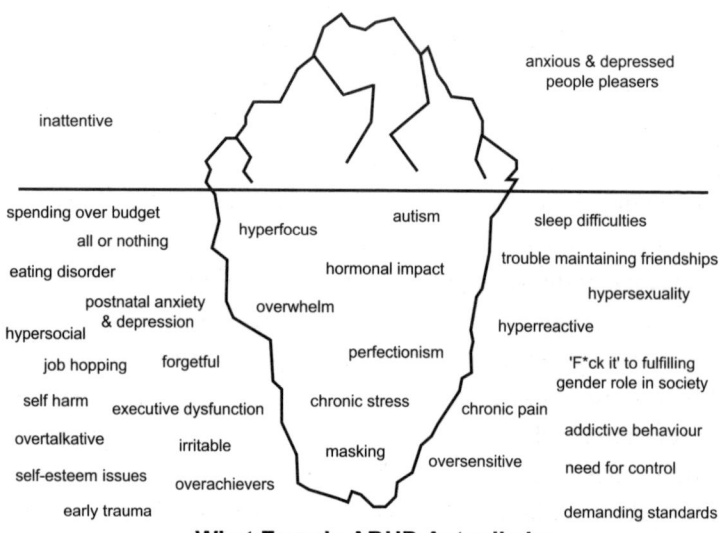

inattentive, anxious and depressed day dreamers and people-pleasers that women with ADHD are often perceived as being.

I initially created a version of this graphic because I grew weary of the ways in which girls and women with ADHD are often described by specialists. It seems as if they're all drawing from the same source passed down by word of mouth, which has ultimately formed our societal beliefs today. Over the years, I've spoken to thousands of women with ADHD around the world and seen first hand how we're an eclectic mix of fire-in-the-belly social justice warriors, both organized and disorganized at different times of our lives. We're creative and really on-top-of-our-sh*t women, who sometimes present in larger-than-life personas yet still often go undetected and unfulfilled, so I knew those sorts of stereotypical descriptions were only scratching the surface.

As the rest of the world only tends to know about the surface stuff – the neurodivergent traits that form the tip of the iceberg – I wrote this book to build on this graphic and uncover the hidden depths below, based on the colourful lives we all lead. The truth is, it wasn't only women who felt underrepresented. Some men with ADHD who also identify as autistic may find that they don't fit neatly into the conventional diagnostic boxes either. Similarly, individuals whose identities intersect with other factors – such as race, gender identity, sexuality or disability – may also experience a sense of exclusion or misrepresentation. My aim is to remind both ourselves and everyone else of our humanity and the areas in which we are more alike than unalike, so we can honour our differences and build a bridge to connect neurodivergent people with the rest of the world.

The book uncovers the nuances of our neurodiverse experiences and humanizes our brain differences based on our generational and genetic stories and eclectic life contexts. It uses science to help make sense of how the places in which we began and live our lives can change the way our neurodivergence and mental health manifest over time. It's an empathetic guide that draws on neuroscience, biology, psychology and sociology, alongside stories from the neurodiversity movement (the social justice movement that seeks equality and inclusion for all neurodivergents), to explain our existential struggles in an inclusive way, so we can find a sense of agency and a toolkit with which to chart our recovery.

I hope you will see me as a compassionate mentor who is learning and healing alongside you, and who has tried everything in this book to give you an empowering lens through which to positively reframe your neurodivergence as you enquire into your past and who you are now.

This is about starting to personalize the way you approach your health so you can hack your neurotype and become the optimum version of yourself – to make the most of this one life of yours, and to spark self-awareness and self-compassion for healing and forgiveness.

I aim to arm you with the words that will enable you to self-advocate to gain acceptance and a sense of belonging, and to stabilize the shake-up that can accompany your enquiry into your neurodivergence label. I hope you will also see me as your protective friend who is there to hold your hand when the world closes in on you, so you can search within, find your voice and bounce right back.

## ADHD AND ME

There's something to be said about carving a career based entirely on your authentic way of being. Some days, it feels as though by understanding how your own mind works, you've solved the puzzle of the human condition. Other days, sharing your story can reveal an uncomfortable truth that unlocks yet another unfathomably dark part of you. When the discovery deepens in the coming weeks, months and years into your later-in-life ADHD diagnosis, at times you wonder if you could just take a break from it and exchange everything you know for the blissful oblivion of yesteryear. The years that, even if they were punctuated by the lowest of lows, also gave you the highest of highs. Even if you were confused about the way you sometimes acted, at least you didn't have to deal with knowing the reason behind why you behaved in the way you did. Because, yes, this realization can be empowering, but it can also be incredibly lonely.

My deep dive into what happened to me and then to the ADHD community collectively began with a very simple but real need to find a place to belong. At the time when I got diagnosed, I found it hard to identify with stories of ADHD alone, and with autism alone. It was only after I was diagnosed with ADHD that I resonated with being autistic too, and four years later, finally received a hard-won diagnosis of autism spectrum disorder.[1] I identified partly with what others said: the bit about not being able to apply yourself, of nearly failing subjects in school. That was until I reached the age of 16, when my life was changed by a wonderful teacher by the name of Mrs Fun, who sparked my love for biology. I lapped up every biology lesson and found comfort in the knowledge that everything in life happens as a process. From where I'm standing now, it helps me understand the evolution of human behaviours, from the genes we inherited to the person you see in front of you today.

When I was growing up in Malaysia, I was a know-it-all in science lessons, but knew nothing at all about social norms and rules. I was the girl whose hand would shoot up into the air to answer a question and I was always up for a debate, and as such, I made very few friends later in university. It didn't matter, because I was focused on one goal only: to achieve good enough grades to secure a scholarship to study abroad and fulfil my dream of doing cancer research.

When I landed on English soil at the age of 23, having received the first Malaysian Prime Minister scholarship to pursue my postgraduate degree in cancer research, I found myself feeling very alone and scared, bawling my eyes out in my tiny room in the residential hall and asking, 'What have I done?' But then I swiftly abandoned the books and started to truly LIVE. I guess it was only to be expected of a young woman who'd been brought up by parents who were simultaneously overprotective and emotionally neglectful. Looking back, my whole life until I left Malaysia had been about studying so I could experience life abroad and run away from prying eyes and stifling Southeast Asian societal expectations. Even if I didn't have the words for it then,

I wanted the freedom to pursue my own truth and what was really important to me.

Unfortunately, my life in England lacked accountability as there was no one to check in on me and I could do whatever I wanted. And in this way, what I now call my 'train wreck' years ensued – a rotation of alcohol-fuelled parties, travel and heartbreak. I was groomed by a man who I eventually submitted a sexual harassment case against, although I didn't initially understand his intentions or how to defend myself from him. Several misadventures later, I found my PhD in jeopardy. When crisis beckoned in the form of a looming thesis deadline, I battened down the hatches and miraculously scraped through, receiving excellent recommendations and a job interview at Harvard.

However, by then my confidence as a scientist had hit rock bottom. So, at the age of 30, and with three degrees in genetics, molecular biology, microbiology, biochemistry and cancer research under my belt, I left the lab to begin again . . . as a writer. My fall from grace was palpable at dinner parties whenever I went back to Malaysia, and I felt deeply lost without my anchor in science. In the years to come, I remained in a relationship that offered me a safe space, while I searched for a career that would light me up, eventually accepting that it was time to embrace motherhood.

My route has been anything but conventional – as is the ADHD way – and a decade later, my ability to connect the dots finally paid off. At the age of 40, soon after my own ADHD diagnosis, I founded ADHD Girls, a social impact company that began with an Instagram account and a YouTube channel. I remember diving into all the research available on women and girls with ADHD and distinctly feeling that we were on the cusp of a societal shift in understanding why ADHD presented differently in women and girls, compared to men and boys.

Straight out of the pandemic, newspapers, magazines and TV channels started to feature interviews with people who'd been diagnosed as adults and who didn't look anything like the ADHD stereotype of the naughty white boy or the character of Sheldon from

*The Big Bang Theory*, with the monotone voice commonly associated with autism. Many of these people were the journalists who write our favourite newspaper columns, celebrities, successful entrepreneurs and also everyday people – women like me, who until the early noughties weren't even included in the research for ADHD.

Because of my cross-cultural background, I was curious to find more people who didn't fully identify with the usual ADHD criteria, people who had somehow soldiered on through school and found a way to cope with neurodivergence, and remained 'hidden' until life became too overwhelming to bear. My Conversations with Women with ADHD campaign amplified the voices of women with ADHD around the world, and I found that despite being united by a common label, the way ADHD manifested for us vastly differed across our varied cultures, races, social classes, co-occurring neurodiverse experiences, life stages and circumstances. My Utopia podcast uncovered hidden stories of neurodivergents from underrepresented groups and amplified diverse voices that weren't initially included in discussions around neurodiversity.

My own story as a cross-cultural neurodivergent woman has helped me see the grey areas others sometimes miss concerning the diversity of our neurodiverse experiences, and my aim in this book is therefore to guide you on how to survive and thrive after your diagnosis, whatever your individual circumstances. Mindful of the fact that ADHD shows up differently in all of us, together we're going to tackle the core issues of your neurodivergence – so that you can tailor personalized strategies to support your own life, moving forward.

## EMPOWERING YOURSELF

Today, there has been a significant increase in the number of people seeking an ADHD diagnosis, with the waiting time for this now being an average of eight years in some parts of the UK.[2] Yet this in turn begs the question why has there been such an upsurge in those seeking diagnosis? And if women have been overlooked in the past, who else might we be missing?

Those of us with ADHD are born with a neurotype that predisposes us to an increased sensitivity to the world, which can be a double-edged sword. Whether our neurodivergence becomes a gift or a hindrance lies in our individual stories – the hand we're dealt in life, our early beginnings, the parents we have, and those serendipitous encounters along the way that shape our life trajectories.

Without a clinician having a detailed knowledge of your own unique neurodiverse experience, it can be incredibly difficult to get diagnosed with the right label and then to make sense of the information associated with that label. Even then, how do you trust that diagnosis, when it's based on the subjective perception of the diagnosing clinician? And how are you to banish a sense of imposter syndrome, even if you've received the diagnosis, given that assessment criteria are biased towards the experiences of a part of the population only? (As we'll see later, the criteria were originally based on studies of young white boys.) Most importantly, after a diagnosis, what are you supposed to do with that information?

There are so many questions, that it can almost feel impossible to know where to begin, which is why it's important to explore the complexity of our human experiences beneath the tip of the neurodivergence iceberg. Because it's what we feel that we usually need the most support with.

Neurodivergence can manifest within a spectrum of experiences across different communities and life circumstances. This is why it's important to accept that whatever your neurodiverse experience is, it is yours and yours only; it's a combination of both nature and nurture, and a culmination of how the life you've experienced has interacted with the genes you inherited. Whether it becomes a strength or a disability varies from person to person and wholly depends on their individual experiences.

Because of this, it matters who and where you learn about neurodivergence from. It can be the difference between reinforcing learned helplessness – the process by which we can learn to feel helpless and powerless in the face of challenging situations – and finding personal empowerment. One will keep you in despair, while the other will activate a mobilizing energy that propels you into hope and a chance at a fulfilling life.

## HOW TO USE THIS BOOK

My hope is that this book will act as an essential resource for anyone who has gone through their whole life feeling confused about how they've behaved, thought or felt, or struggled with their mental health. Alongside personal insights, the science that underpins this book can offer a sense of cohesion, because once we can explain what happens in our bodies and brains when we interact with our environment – which gives rise to our neurodivergent behaviours – this can spark self-understanding, forgiveness and enable us to self-advocate and form more authentic relationships.

This book takes a deep dive to explore the hidden layers of the ADHD iceberg.

**Step 1** looks at the life-changing experience of getting a diagnosis of ADHD in adulthood. It considers the double-edged sword of diagnostic labels and casts light on how neurodivergence is often pathologized in medical journals, yet what makes us 'bad' from some perspectives is precisely what makes us good in different circumstances. This chapter also tackles the sense of shame that can arise on receiving a diagnosis.

**Step 2** unpacks the co-occurring conditions that accompany some of the most common neurodiverse experiences, whether these travel together from the genes passed down our lineage or emerge as a result of our unfolding lives, and the spectrum in which they manifest based on what is innate and how we adapted to life in society.

**Step 3** introduces the delicate balance of nature versus nurture in influencing how our ADHD impacts us and manifests itself in our lives. It helps us understand what is different about the way we're wired from a genetic and biological perspective, so we can identify our own personal needs. It also looks at common physical health conditions in the collective community, as although we might not be affected by them ourselves, an awareness of them means we will be better placed to cope, should they arise.

**Step 4** considers how genes naturally evolve and the ways in which our neurodiversity is also influenced by our environment and upbringing. It considers how the ways in which our neurodiversity expresses itself is shaped by our families, cultural norms, beliefs and rules, gender and our environment, and how we can move forward with this knowledge to instil a positive sense of identity in ourselves.

**Step 5** examines the biggest emotional needs for neurodivergent individuals and illustrates the gradual evolution of our emotional landscape from our brain structure and chemistry, nervous system, and the life we've lived. It looks at common themes in the neurodiverse community around rejection sensitivity dysphoria (RSD), trauma, sensory needs, affective empathy, socio-communication differences, alexithymia (also known as emotional blindness) and dyslexithymia (the struggle to express feelings).

**Step 6** explores our changing relationships as our traits come into sharp focus, when we question who we are and where our coping strategies begin. You may feel the need to unmask in your closest relationships (to strip away those behaviours you've adopted in an attempt to 'fit in'), and thus have a greater need to be understood and feel safe, to dismantle your old life and rebuild a new authentic you. This chapter will give you tangible strategies to navigate this transition and the tools to communicate in different relationships. It also looks at common issues in neurodivergent relationships and considers the role of personality disorders.

**Step 7** focuses on neurodiversity at work, depicting the common challenges neurodivergent individuals face. It also provides best practices around navigating performance feedback and perceived criticisms, and how to communicate your needs to your managers and colleagues so you don't shoot yourself in the foot. In addition, this chapter integrates different life contexts in the workplace.

**Step 8** is about the importance of connecting with your community and finding comfort in like-minded connections. It also addresses what our individual preferences may be when it comes to connecting with others. This chapter looks at how we can be a part of the change to support others and educate society about the nuances of our experiences – to banish stigma and create a world that recognizes neurodivergence as a shared humanity.

**Step 9** brings it all together and will cast light on your new day-to-day life in motion. It illuminates how your social environment can present structure, routine and wellness, but also stressors and triggers that intricately impact your mind and body, and shape how you show up. This chapter addresses how to apply all that you have learned so far in your quest for self-mastery, integrating this into your daily interactions with the people and events in your life that shape your unique reality.

As you go through these steps and join me on this journey, my hope is that you will also go through a metamorphosis, which needs to follow its own rhythm and time. I hope you will see that every past misadventure in your life held a valuable lesson within it; every brave and spontaneous decision represented an area in which you needed to grow; every heartbreak taught you to treat yourself and others gently; and every career pivot honed the skills you needed to discover a purpose that will eventually help you break out of the fortress you created to contain your infinite imagination, wild heart and free spirit. It's time to excavate the hidden layers of the ADHD iceberg.

# Step I:
# Understand It's Not Your Fault

In Step 1, we are going to be looking at how receiving a diagnosis is the very tip of the ADHD iceberg. Alongside helping you make sense of your past, a diagnosis can also entail questioning your understanding of yourself as you come to terms with the label that you've acquired and its significance. Moreover, diagnostic labels themselves aren't completely straightforward and might not capture the nuances of your experience – which is why it's so important to consider the whole picture and to explore the hidden layers of the ADHD iceberg.

## THE DAY YOU GET A DIAGNOSIS

At this first stage of exploring the ADHD iceberg, you may be grappling with a diagnosis or the possibility of one, and you probably still have many more questions than answers. If you've already walked out of an ADHD assessment with a diagnosis, very likely at an older age than you expected to be, you may have been engulfed by the enormity of the label you just acquired. I'm guessing that you may have felt relieved and elated at first. And then . . . a tad battered. Drained. Confused. As though you've just aced an exam, but it took some re-traumatizing to do it.

The doctors needed to know precisely how your ADHD 'reduces the quality of social, academic or occupational functioning' to grant you the diagnosis. So, you've had to strip back your masks – those layers of learned behaviours you've presented to the world since childhood – and regurgitate every harrowing detail of your life. The world is still fed a diet of stigmatizing and outdated beliefs about ADHD and co-occurring conditions like autism. Depending on who you see to get assessed, that healthcare professional may be drawing on a medicalized model of psychiatry that is steeped in the traditional roles of the 'therapist' (who fixes) and the 'patient' (who is in need of fixing, a label that I personally don't agree with in this instance; hence why I use quotation marks throughout for this word) – a relationship that may even cause feelings of powerlessness to resurface for you.

Upon leaving the assessment with a diagnosis, there are now a number of things you're aware you should do, although your head is still spinning. If you've adopted the label of ADHD for yourself long before receiving a formal diagnosis, it now feels even more real. First, you need to go home and break the news to your friends and family. You're still grappling with how you feel yourself, so how on earth will you relay these emotions to others? Will they understand? Or will they begin to see you as a liability? And is this experience unique to you and your family, or are other people going through the same process too?

Somewhere within yourself, you may wonder whether it's all your fault. 'Did I get this from my parents or am I just the unlucky one? Did I pass this on to my kids? Is this something that will persist throughout my and their lives?'

Back out in the world, you're the same, yet you're suddenly changed in more ways than you can imagine. You must now learn to explain the reasons behind every minute detail of your behaviour to help others understand you, but whether or not they will, is something you can't really control.

If you're employed, you could go through a process where you use your new diagnosis to explain why you need support at work; however, some 70 per cent of neurodivergents don't open up about their diagnosis to their employer.[1] Why would we, when we are saddled with the responsibility of a prevailing stigma against neurodivergence?

It can all feel so overwhelming.

'Who even am I?' I hear you ask.

In a sense, you are unravelling. We usually think of this process as being negative, but actually all it means is that you're now being forced to shed all the layers that became your armour, because they no longer serve you. Somewhere within, there are parts of you that feel imprisoned, misunderstood and neglected. All of these parts want to break free.

It's time to begin to dig deeper for the answers to explain what has happened to you and others like you, who have been overlooked until now. You have now been given a diagnostic label you can present to yourself and others – but what is underneath it? What is informing it? This stage is just the tip of the ADHD iceberg.

### What Behaviours Are Associated with ADHD?

There are some collective challenges we face as neurodivergents that can manifest as the following behaviours:

- Scatter-brained and always multi-tasking
- Suffering from stress, burnout, fatigue and overwhelm
- Executive function challenges
- Heightened fight-or-flight response
- Depression
- Anxiety and panic attacks
- Temper outbursts that come like a tsunami and leave us feeling ashamed in the aftermath
- Emotional dysregulation
- Aches and pains
- Sleep difficulties
- Mood challenges during monthly menstrual cycles and large hormonal transitions
- Addictive behaviours – coping with alcohol, drugs, sugar or sex
- Mental and emotional health challenges

- Multiple personality traits at different times of the day, week and month, depending on the presence of triggers or glimmers
- Rejection sensitivity dysphoria (RSD) – where perceived rejection causes intense emotional pain and dysregulation
- Repeating patterns of behaviour that compromise relationships
- Feeling misunderstood and ostracized
- Low self-esteem
- Highly controlling
- Holding high standards to others and being a perfectionist ourselves
- Job hopping and poor financial control
- Not wanting to be with others, but feeling lonely alone

As we will see in Steps 3 and 4, you may experience some, none or quite a few of these traits at different times and stages of your life. A lot depends on your personal physiology, upbringing and life circumstances.

## THE PROS AND CONS OF LABELS

Within the neurodiverse community, there are different views about neurodivergence labels. Some of us feel a sense of relief at finally getting a diagnostic label that explains our way of being, others may challenge the necessity of labels altogether, while yet others have views on them that change over time.

When you are diagnosed later in life, labels can be useful in some ways. A label can help change your life for the better and, in some cases, it may even be important for your survival. Yet this is where things can turn on their head. While a label can free you in some ways, it can also hold you hostage.

## STEP I: UNDERSTAND IT'S NOT YOUR FAULT

| PROS | CONS |
|---|---|
| A label can help you make sense of who you are, understand your challenges, validate the distressing experiences you've had, lessen the shame and guilt that you've felt, and make you feel understood. | Getting diagnosed with a neurodevelopmental or mental health label singles us out as different. |
| A diagnosis can provide a starting point for you to understand how to work with your mind better, foster self-forgiveness, self-compassion, and look for the support you need. | If we label a trait as bad so we can fix it, we risk ignoring the fact that all our personality traits lie on a spectrum and that we are multi-dimensional human beings. |
| It can afford you access to a community of people with whom you perhaps share parallel experiences and give you a sense of belonging. | Labels don't come about in isolation but can be influenced by a number of factors, not least the culture and gendered expectations of those who define them and agree upon them, which can be subjective and limiting. |
| In some countries like the UK and the US, a neurodivergence label is required to access funding and resources via the healthcare, education, workplace and welfare systems. | In acquiring a label, we may find ourselves trying to squeeze ourselves into a box that wasn't originally made with us in mind, and that might not be at all comfortable. |

## WHY WERE WE MISSED?

When we go looking for an ADHD diagnosis, many of us don't expect to walk ourselves into a major life event, where we find ourselves asking, 'Why were we missed?' Why did it take so long for medical professionals to confirm our own suspicions, and for us to be able to get the understanding and support we need? We may begin to examine every aspect of our lives to figure out where it all went wrong, and where it could have gone better. Today, there is an unprecedented demand for answers, a collective deep dive, unveiling a lost generation of people who've had to navigate their neurodivergence journey on their own.

Along the way, many women who've been diagnosed in later life have realized that they seem to share striking commonality with non-neurodivergent women, so much so that the latter have found themselves questioning if they have ADHD too, due to the blinding similarities in our daily lives, such as feeling overwhelmed, experiencing negative internal thoughts, and emotional dysregulation from having to juggle it all.

There are many hidden stories like these beneath the surface of the iceberg, involving so much more than genes and neuroscience, such as how our lives in society shape the expression of our behaviours. For example, young girls are expected to carry the female generational burden. If they fail to fulfil that role in the eyes of their parents, partners, their children and society, they may internalize that sense of failure – to their own detriment. The situation can be further complicated when girls and women receive a diagnosis such as ADHD, which of course has a history of its own.

## A SHORT HISTORY OF ADHD DIAGNOSES

In terms of how we feel about an ADHD diagnosis ourselves, much depends on what those around us know about the label, the stigma that arises from the public not fully understanding its nuances, and how that might affect us. While public understanding of neurodivergence labels is changing for the better today, women in particular are still affected by the consequences of years of underrepresentation in the medical system.

This is particularly evident in the history of ADHD diagnosis in children. Back in 1902, British paediatrician Sir George Still observed 'an abnormal defect of moral control in children', whereby affected children were unable to control their behaviour in the same way a typical child would.[2] The traits he observed were:

- Inability to control impulses
- Disruptive or oppositional behaviour
- Hyperactivity or excessive movement
- Difficulty in conforming to social norms

These children were still intelligent, he helpfully remarked. But bear in mind he was only referring to boys and the behaviours he focused on were externalized – loud, visible and disruptive.

If research and psychiatry is based mainly on the experiences of men and boys in Western culture, then how are women and girls, and people from different cultures, race, sexual orientations and social classes meant to find the answers they are looking for about their neurodivergence? Especially if many of our traits tend to be internalized, socialized and variable in accordance with our cultural or racial norms?

It wasn't until 1997 that truly meaningful research was finally carried out into girls with ADHD, when Professor Stephen Hinshaw, Professor of Psychiatry and Behavioural Sciences at the University of California, carried out the largest foundational study on girls with ADHD, the Berkeley Girls with ADHD Longitudinal Study.[3] Hinshaw followed the development of girls with ADHD from the average age of nine to twenty-six, and discovered that girls and boys show broadly similar presentations but differ largely in their outcome. While this marked the start of addressing the gender gap in ADHD, it was still missing the voices of other underrepresented groups.

Alongside many women today opening up about the mental health challenges they face as neurodivergent individuals, while fulfilling the role of females in society, we have witnessed rising ADHD and autism diagnoses in recent years. Data from Clinical Partners, a UK mental healthcare and diagnostics provider, recorded an estimated 254,400 women took an online test for ADHD in 2022, a 3,200 per cent increase from 2019.[4]

We can also see these limitations when looking at autism diagnoses; for example, a population-based study in the UK showed an exponential 787 per cent increase in those being diagnosed with autism in the last two decades.[5] While this data looks like a big increase, the general spread of the population in that study is broad in terms of gender and social status, so there's no way of knowing if this includes underrepresented identities. A recent study by paediatrician Dr Robert McCrossin showed that 80 per cent of autistic girls remain undiagnosed by the age of 18, which has been attributed to a combination of clinician bias, high masking (adopting an acceptable appearance in an attempt to fit in), misdiagnoses and difference in presentations compared to autistic boys and men.[6]

Cue the new millennium, and adults everywhere who have been diagnosed with ADHD find themselves carrying the burden of the outdated perception of the label. It seems we cannot accept the validation that comes from a diagnosis without also accepting the burden of a label. To be an ADHDer is to carry stigmatized beliefs about naughty white boys. While our understanding of ADHD has evolved from one of hyperactivity, impulsivity and distractibility to one that concerns emotional dysregulation and executive dysfunction, it still seems very simplistic. Is it a given that we all struggle with our day-to-day lives and are we all emotional hot messes? Where is the wider context?

## Who Defines a Label Like ADHD Today?

Depending on which country you reside in, your mental health and medical professionals may refer to the *Diagnostic and Statistical*

*Manual of Mental Disorders* (DSM-5 and DSM-5-TR), the *International Classification of Diseases* (ICD-11), neurodivergence-specific rating scales, and country-specific clinical guidelines when trying to assess you for a neurodevelopmental and/or mental health condition.

The ICD-11 (11th version) was developed by a global collaboration of over 300 specialists across 55 countries and published by the World Health Organization (WHO) in 2019. The ICD-11 covers clinical diagnoses for illnesses of the mind and body, and is more accessible than the DSM-5, as it's available to all and open to the public for submissions.[7]

The DSM-5-TR (text revision) is the 2022 revised edition of DSM-5, developed by the American Psychiatric Association (APA), with a task force that oversees work groups comprising of mental health and medical professionals from prestigious academic and mental health institutions *'around the world'*.

Here's the catch. The criteria within each label in the DSM that psychiatrists and mental health professionals use to determine (very subjectively) whether you get diagnosed or not were derived via a *consensus* from discussions within this elite circle – *not* through objective laboratory measures.

Let's consider who's at that table, having those discussions. The DSM-5-TR was defined by a consensus consisting of 21 per cent of international experts, as compared to about 30 per cent of them in DSM-5 (in 2013).[8] So, in referring to contributing experts from *'around the world'*, they mean only 21 per cent of all international experts.

Working in the field of neurodiversity, I've been in rooms where, as a Southeast Asian woman, I'm in the minority. These rooms are often full of people from the dominant culture. The agenda is frequently set by the privileged group and whoever else has a voice. The discussions will thus often cater to the majority. In essence, the priority is often given to those who speak up and even then, the loudest voice tends to lead.

Furthermore, in a project in which psychiatrists are most heavily represented, followed by psychologists and other health professionals (approximately 60 per cent of contributors are psychiatrists, 25 per cent psychologists and 15 per cent other health professionals in the DSM-5-TR), we are going to get a skewed perspective towards seeing mental health issues and neurodivergence as diseases that need treatment.

While both ICD-11 and DSM-5-TR have given more cultural nuance to the development of mental illness, the former is based on an approach that is better at capturing the fluidity of illnesses over time. However, even this has been met with criticism, because medical professionals struggle to differentiate traits such as those associated with ADHD and autism from other mental health disorders, for example. I think this is largely down to the fact that psychiatrists struggle to ask the right questions to get to the answers they need. Indeed, how could they, if they've never walked in our shoes?

The DSM-5-TR has also adopted a more culturally sensitive approach to mental health. Within Section III, clinicians can find a 'Cultural Formulation' section which contains the 'Cultural Formulation Interview (CFI)', a tool for assessing the impact of cultural factors on somebody's clinical presentation and experience. The interview covers four key domains:

> **Domain 1:**
> Cultural definition of the problem: how the individual perceives and describes their mental health issue within their cultural context.

▼

> **Domain 2:**
> Cultural perceptions of cause, context and support: includes beliefs about the cause of the problem, contributing factors and available support systems, including cultural identity.

▼

> **Domain 3:**
> Cultural factors that affect self-coping and past help seeking: examines personal coping strategies and past experiences with seeking help, including barriers faced.

▽

> **Domain 4:**
> Cultural factors that affect current help seeking: explores cultural influences on the individual's willingness and ability to seek professional help at present.

This seems promising. However, it's thought by some to be 'shallow because what is presented as "culture" [...] is too focused on meaning and not enough on practice'.[9] In other words, it's good at describing ideas but fails to describe the reality of living with concrete 'things' in culturally diverse environments.

The fact is, in a country where the majority of clinicians use rating scales to assess conditions like neurodivergence, the DSM-5 can only be used as a reference point, and the presence or lack of cultural sensitivity may very well depend on the assessing clinician's background and personal interests, rather than being based on any formal training on how to apply an intersectional lens to diagnosis and support. The DSM-5 largely divides our challenges into distinct categories in a way that discounts the nuances of our experiences, too; it also neglects to cater for the differences in how we express ourselves when faced with real-world challenges. Most importantly, it doesn't take into account how our neurodiverse experiences change across our lifespan.

In the context of neurodivergence, the labels of ADHD and autism within psychiatric manuals tend to focus on the symptoms that cause major inconveniences to others, reduce our quality of life, or require varying degrees of support. Many of the symptoms listed in the manuals are stereotypical traits such as being overtly hyperactive or impulsive as an ADHDer, or having repeated and restrictive interests and behaviours as an autistic individual, for example.

The more we display these stereotypical symptoms, the more likely we are to be diagnosed with the label. In contrast, less obvious traits such as fatigue, emotional dysregulation or internalized anxiety in high-masking people aren't necessarily covered in this sort of assessment.

And what happens when our experiences diverge from the common stereotypes altogether?

## LABELS AND CULTURAL DIFFERENCES

The diversity in our neurodiverse experiences is two pronged – subject to our individual biology, and to our interactions with the environment. However, the dominant discourse surrounding neurodivergence is still based on biological explanations of cognitive functioning, which is thought to be reflected in behaviours.[10] The DSM-5 posits that 'symptoms must be present in the early developmental period (but may not become fully manifest until social demands exceed limited capacities or may be masked by learned strategies in later life).' But development itself means a process in which our form unfolds in reaction to internal genetic programming, and our biology's interaction with our lives within cultural- and context-dependent rules.

Based on my own experience, I would suggest that instead of displaying anxiety, hyperactivity or impulsivity, someone like me who grew up in a Southeast Asian culture that traditionally values subservience and conformity, for example, would go to great lengths to repress their natural feelings and manifest their neurodivergence as perfectionist tendencies with a high need for control. In my case, over time, this even resulted in a heart condition.

As the psychiatric manuals are developed in the US and Europe, but used by everyone in the world, the need for training around cultural contexts is pivotal. The fact is that culture is not static. It consists of a set of beliefs, practices and ways of life that are passed down from one generation to another; it includes language, religion, family traditions, life stages, ceremonies and rules – and it is always evolving and changing.

Today, many people are influenced by multiple cultures, which help shape their identities and how they understand the world around them. Our unique cultural backgrounds, ethnicity, race and social status influence the following things:

- How we show and experience symptoms used for diagnosis
- Our mental health
- How our experiences, traits and behaviours compare to cultural norms, and our ability to adapt to the surrounding culture
- Our ability to access resources
- The possibility of being exposed to real world challenges that can impact our mental health.

A diagnostic assessment can be challenging when the clinician is using the DSM-5 classification to evaluate an individual from a different ethnic or cultural group, but is unfamiliar with the nuances of that individual's cultural frame of reference. The clinician may also have to contend with their own unconscious bias and beliefs, based on their own background and the window through which they see the world. There is therefore a very real need for cultural training for physicians, because as the situation stands, the system often overlooks people from the underrepresented groups in a particular culture.

All said, neurodivergence and mental health labels don't currently allow for how our individual lives and the society in which we live shape our physical, mental, spiritual and social health. If your experiences don't fit the common diagnostic stereotype, and someone with your beginnings, background and current life circumstances wasn't represented at the table when the consensus about that stereotype was reached, then how could they understand the series of twists and turns that led you here?

You are very likely to be overlooked, misunderstood, misdiagnosed, and perhaps even mistreated – especially if you're a person from the global majority (i.e., those racialized as minorities in white-majority countries but who make up the majority of the world's population), a woman, identify as a different gender from which you were born, have lived across different cultures, or grew up deprived or are currently living without much support. At best, what a psychiatrist will see is a snapshot of your current life on the day you find yourself in their office.

This is where it can be so hard to accept the way professionals and medical journal articles approach a label like ADHD. Even if it helps illuminate an aspect of your neurodivergence, you likely intuitively know it isn't the full picture of YOU. As world-renowned expert on traumatic stress Bessel van der Kolk explores in his book *The Body Keeps the Score*, we cannot ignore the relationships and interactions we had when we were young and how we became the person we are, which requires understanding of our process, a step-by-step evolution of our orientation, capacities and behaviours. The explanation of any diagnosis, especially one such as ADHD, needs to encompass the diversity of who we are, which is influenced by our individual upbringing, life circumstances and the society around us.

## ADHD AND CO-OCCURING CONDITIONS

In acquiring a diagnostic label and opening up to others about it, we may form an allegiance of some sort or another with whichever community shares the same label(s). And that is perfectly okay if the people who're part of this community also share your experiences – from the moment you were born until you got here. But what if your experiences don't fit the mould in ways besides those of culture and gender?

You know who you are better than anyone else does, and you might resonate with some of the traits within an ADHD label, but not all. You may also feel like you resonate with other labels, which taken together, explain you better. Perhaps you're not just an ADHDer, but also identify with being autistic, dyspraxic (having difficulties with coordination and motor skills) or dyslexic (experiencing challenges with reading, writing, or processing language) or are prone to anxiety and depression? As we will see in Step 2, you may even find that these traits present as a continuum, not fully manifested in either a destructive or helpful manner, until you hit challenges in your life that make it hard for you to cope.

If we identify with other types of neurodivergence besides ADHD, how can one neat label ever capture this or reflect the complexity of our personality and experiences? To add to the complexity, late ADHD and autism diagnoses are often accompanied by mental health challenges that have at their root the impact of trauma. The report 'An Asset not a Problem', based on a survey of more than 2,000 university applicants in Bristol, UK, found that autistic and ADHD applicants were more likely to have mental health challenges, 52 per cent had experienced depression recently, and 63 per cent had experienced anxiety in the last two years – both statistics being above the average for all applicants. The report also found that neurodivergent applicants were also more likely to have experienced obsessive compulsive disorder (OCD), eating disorders, personality disorders and post-traumatic stress disorder (PTSD).[11]

Trauma colours the lens through which we see the world, so it can be challenging to verbalize to clinicians why we feel or act a certain way when we struggle to understand it ourselves. If trauma causes disintegration within the self, then how are we to communicate succinctly what we felt and experienced – especially when the assessment process itself can feel disempowering and re-traumatizing?

We need to remember that the nervous system is sensitive to life changes, when the challenges we face exceed our abilities to cope with them. Milestones such as starting university in a city far away from family support, getting married or becoming a new parent, divorce, bereavement and increasing care-giving responsibilities can contribute to persistent chronic stress. Without adequate support, we can experience mental and emotional distress that create the perfect storm which may finally lead to the discovery of our neurodivergence label.

## HOW DO YOU FEEL ABOUT AN ADHD LABEL?

We have to see ourselves as a *whole*, the sum of all our parts, to be empowered to drive our recovery by asking the right questions, rather than taking the passive and disempowered role of the 'patient'. As a starting point, understanding what the label means to you personally, being empowered with self-knowledge, and seeking a professional who understands your unique individuality can make the difference between making progress in your journey and being further stigmatized.

Research prior to 2013 (when the diagnostic criteria became more relaxed) seemed to suggest that when someone learns they have ADHD, their sense of negativity towards themselves automatically increases.[12] This was no doubt due to the stigma associated with the condition, partially enabled by the medical community itself, as we've seen. In contrast, it's a bit more of a mixed picture today, partly due to the neurodiverse community itself, whose voices are beginning to make themselves heard, demanding that the labels reflect who we are.

As women aged between 23 and 49 are the largest group contributing to the rise in adult ADHD diagnoses today, with figures nearly doubling from 2020 to 2022,[13] it's particularly interesting to hear what they have to say about this. Many women interviewed in recent studies expressed feelings of relief and self-acceptance from a late diagnosis, having spent decades none the wiser about the way their minds work and having experienced significant challenges in their relationships, especially if they became mothers.[14] However, they also felt trepidation around not knowing how other people would react to this news or how to discuss it with their loved ones and colleagues without inviting stigma or, worse, infantilization, causing them to internalize problems which then caused them further challenges. It's not easy, for example, to explain your experiences to your workplace occupational health assessor when they try to determine your workplace needs, which are considered only from the point of view that you have ADHD. What about the rest of your life that ADHD affects, the parts that are constantly on fire from trying to juggle everything?

At this particular stage of your life, you may even feel as if you are going through a grieving process, where everything feels more intense than usual (see Step 6, page 184, for more on the grief cycle). You may be particularly sensitive to the ways in which medical and other professionals speak about labels like ADHD, which can sometimes unknowingly perpetuate a negative emotional contagion in a community that is likely to suffer from mental and emotional distress akin to post-traumatic stress disorder during significant life transitions such as this.[15] Members of this community need sufficient light to make sense of the darkness. We need some good news, and a balanced perspective of our unique strengths and abilities, based on the individual stories of our lives.

Above all, when we see our neurodivergence as the central controlling narrative in our lives and we accept its documented challenges at face value, we may lose the capacity to reinvent ourselves. And we risk remaining stuck in the very place we've been trying to escape from our whole lives. So what are our options?

## TREATMENT OPTIONS

If you're lucky enough to receive a diagnosis, your professional will refer to yet another set of guidelines that decide how to devise your treatment. These guidelines are based on what the medical community understand about neurodivergence and mental health currently, and how quickly we managed to get this integrated into the healthcare system.

Based on these guidelines, you may be given a couple of treatment options. The first option could be to trial a medication and start a course of a heavily stigmatized class-B drug, a pretty radical thought. Perhaps you've never taken anything stronger than paracetamol or ibuprofen in your life. When it concerns ADHD, not everyone is going to benefit from taking stimulant medication, and even when our traits are helped by taking them, we need to question which neurobiological pathway it's really supporting and whether focusing on increasing the levels of neurotransmitters could affect other downstream or parallel biochemical pathways in our brains and body systems.

In the UK, another option may be therapy on the NHS. You may have seen TV shows depicting therapy sessions, where patients unpick every detail of their lives with insightful professionals, seemingly uninhibited. In reality, these sessions will probably be far more structured. They will be less focused on a free-flow 'talk therapy' and more on cognitive behavioural therapy (CBT), which involves reprogramming the ways you approach a situation here and now, rather than dealing with how your past affects your current patterns.

CBT dissects present challenges by looking into the links between how we think and feel influences how we behave. It is said to help those with depression, anxiety and obsessive compulsive disorder (OCD). Conventional CBT can work well for those who are going through the motions, unaware of the reasons behind their behaviours, and who are generally good at doing as they're told. However, in reality it might not be the most useful therapy at a time when you're still unpacking what your diagnosis means for you or if your neurodivergence means that, like me, you have a pathological demand avoidance aka persistent drive for autonomy (PDA) profile. When standard CBT is used in a session, your inner voice may even say a resounding 'No!' – even more so when you've masked your condition for so long and want to now exert your autonomy, but don't yet know how to start. (See Step 5, for more on starting therapy.)

Frankly, as a cross-cultural woman who was raised in Asia but 'grew up' in the UK, therapy still feels extremely privileged to me. I'd never in my wildest dreams imagined that in my forties, I would pay someone to unpack the ways I'd been traumatized in childhood. Looking back in therapy and connecting the dots was extremely painful to do, because the memories started to resurface in my daily life, along with feelings of shame.

To complicate matters further, the current limitations of diagnostic labels, which don't take into account the full picture of who we are, point to the unreliability of using a label to devise a holistic treatment plan. In 2010, the National Institute of Mental Health (NIMH) recognized this lack of diagnostic and treatment precision in psychiatry and devised a project to research mental health conditions, called the Research Domain Criteria (RDoC).[16] This ground-breaking project focused on studying biological pathways that underpin the manifestation of behavioural traits across the general population. The RDoC aims to address the symptom heterogeneity seen in mental disorders through bringing together genetics, neuroscience and behavioural science and casting light on how our life in society affects our biology. As the RDoC framework continues to evolve and influence research trajectories and contemporary psychiatric studies, it remains an integral part of the NIMH's strategy to advance the understanding and treatment of mental health conditions through a multi-dimensional and integrative research approach.

When the system's inherent focus is to treat people so they are well enough to be productive members of society without looking at what they need to become *wholly* well, how can someone like you and I ever hope to find a path to recovery?

Well, we can begin by doing our own research. And a powerful place to start is by getting to know ourselves better, which entails exploring the different layers of the ADHD iceberg.

## DIGGING DEEPER AFTER A DIAGNOSIS

As we start to navigate the new sense of identity that can accompany a diagnosis, our traits can come into sharp focus. While this may validate our previous struggles, it can also make us fixate on those traits that are associated with a label such as ADHD to the extent that, over time, we may start to think that is all we are and feel a little lost. Just *who are we* underneath the mask that we've been wearing for all these years?

However, unmasking is less about revealing the person behind the mask and highlighting the traits that make you struggle, and more of an excavation into the layers that make you who you are. Herein lies your story. It's about the deeper layers that aren't initially revealed upon your diagnosis. The layers may seem confusing at first, and sometimes even appear to be at war with one another, yet they hold the key to unlocking the wholeness of your way of being. In this book, we're going to set out on a journey to explore these layers of the ADHD iceberg stage by stage together.

The thing about being diagnosed later in life is that, yes, we may need to dismantle our lives now to figure out who we are, but we also need to remember that no part of our life has been wasted. Every experience has given us the chance to find our own way, create the strategies that got us here (whether good or maladaptive ones), and made us resilient. These may be in equal parts beautiful and tragic, but the beautiful parts still exist, and enlightenment can come from sharing the lessons afforded by our tragedies.

Moreover, in dismantling who we are, parts inside ourselves will be shaken up, bringing to the fore our dormant motivations, desires, needs and wants in our relationships. Then we can look at the hand we've been dealt, embrace the 'bad' parts with the 'good' parts, and decide, 'What kind of life do I want? One that continues to put me in the passenger seat of my life or the one where I dare to climb back into the driver's seat?' However, it's important to be aware that opening up to ourselves in this way can also mean tackling some uncomfortable feelings, especially at first.

**Reflection**
Take a moment now to consider how you feel about ADHD in relation to yourself. Do those feelings take any particular form or even manifest themselves in your body in any way? What might help you to process your feelings – a quiet activity like journaling or physical exercise such as running or walking?

## FACING SHAME

A key thing to realize is that if you're not careful about how you see a label, you can easily internalize a sense of stigma around it. This can be confusing, especially when you may feel that you're supposed to feel more empowered and driven to speak about your authentic needs after having received a diagnosis. I remember, too, the shame that I felt when I started to unpack the things that had happened to me. About those times I never said 'no' louder. About how I could never seem to hold a firm boundary as an adult . . . And it all hit me again. Somehow, I felt responsible. I know I'm not alone in feeling like this.

A sense of stigma following a diagnosis such as ADHD can affect your self-esteem and make you forget about the things you could easily do before diagnosis. It may even rip away the coping strategies you created. You will likely go through the process of associating with your challenges, at first, more than your strengths. But you will also come to understand that associating with your strengths is what got you through the difficult times.

And your eyes will start to open to the fact that despite being connected to others by a condition that has become your way of being, you're nevertheless a unique individual. You are the sum of nature and nurture. In addition to your neurological differences, you are the sum of your beginnings, your culture, your relationships and the people and events that influenced you. There is so much more to you than a label, stigmatizing or otherwise. When you get diagnosed later in life, while you may feel that your life afterwards is significantly worse than your life before, at least for a while, you have to realize that blaming yourself is like blaming evolution.

You need to remember that internalizing limiting beliefs about yourself can keep you in victim mode, when you are anything but. You *can* overcome this and develop a new mindset in which you radically accept who you are, balancing your will and being realistic about your needs. I know how hard this is, but you have to let go of the shame and reframe any negative feelings you have about your neurodivergence.

However, tackling our individual feelings of shame can be complicated by the attitudes of society itself. With the media sensationalizing diagnoses of ADHD and autism, we are faced with a rhetorical question – is it a trend? This sort of questioning and self-doubt can be harmful to neurodivergents who may be trying to resolve years of shame and guilt attached to events in their lives.

Listening to negative narratives about our way of being can be damaging as it reinforces feelings of learned helplessness. It can make us feel vulnerable. You may even find yourself questioning whether you're truly neurodivergent or whether the traits you show are a result of your upbringing. I don't blame you for feeling like this. I've internalized a lot of the negative narratives on ADHD and autism myself. In fact, the research suggests that by the age of 12, a child with ADHD has internalized 20,000 negative messages.[17] I guess we are all in some ways dealing with some level of pain.

Equipped with this insight, it's important that we don't take everything we read about neurodiversity as gospel – especially as the internet is laden with hundreds of thousands of pathologizing medical journals. And I should know, because I've read them in order to write this book for you! (You're welcome.) Instead, we can begin to reframe the negative messages we've received over the years, beginning right now.

| COMMON NEGATIVE MESSAGE | POSITIVE REFRAME |
| --- | --- |
| Why are you so restless? | Your energy is powerful – let's find ways to channel it into things you enjoy |
| You are so sensitive | You're incredibly perceptive to what's going on around you |
| You never listen | I notice you process information differently – how can I help support your focus? |
| You are too intense/too much | Your passion is a gift, never shrink it to fit someone else's comfort |
| You are lazy/not trying hard enough | I see how hard you're trying – let's explore ways that work for your brain |
| You are always forgetting things | Your brain is busy with big ideas, let's find systems that work for you |
| Why can't you be more like X? | You are wonderfully *you* – and the world needs exactly that |

## MOVING ON FROM STIGMA TO SELF-KNOWLEDGE

So how then do we move forward, when it seems the current discourse around neurodiversity appears to be broadly divided into challenges versus superpowers? And is neurodivergence actually a superpower?

In my experience, it's only a superpower if we can wield the power within our strengths without this also affecting the quality of our life and those we care for. Instead, we can begin to move forward by getting curious about who we truly are. To understand the contexts in which our neurodivergence influences how we individually show up in past and present contexts. And to process any shame and guilt that surface.

## Take a Moment to Meet Yourself, Here and Now

To start the process of freeing yourself from the shackles of shame and reconnecting with your neurodivergent strengths, I'd like you to take a moment to reflect on your feelings about a diagnosis of neurodiversity. You might want to journal about this, so you can come back to it later.

1. Do a mental scan of your body. Do you have any aches or pains? Any discomfort or cramps, for example? What, if any, emotion do you associate with this?
2. Notice and observe any sensations of fear or shame without judgement, seeing them as just sensations in the body.
3. Become curious about the feelings and where they come from, exploring any ideals or expectations that may be causing them. Recognize how much of it was contributed by your social conditioning and rules. (Conditioning refers to a learning process that shapes our behaviours and emotions. This often happens unconsciously.)
4. Can you loosen attachment to the ideals causing fear or shame by questioning their helpfulness and origin, or even imagine life without them?
5. How does this suggestion make you feel?

### YOUR STORY

Self-awareness is a gift that keeps on giving in every relationship we navigate in life. And when we can start to develop self-awareness without judgement, we move another step closer to embracing a new perspective free from fear or shame, and to moving through the world with trust, confidence and self-love.

As our neurodiverse experiences are so diverse, to understand our unique experiences, we need to reframe the traits we read about in relation to things like ADHD and autism and view them through the lens of our individual realities. To know ourselves is to know that we are multi-layered. As the ancient Greek philosopher Aristotle wrote in *Metaphysics*, 'The whole is greater than the sum of its parts.' The sum of our parts lies beyond the surface of what others can see at the very tip of the ADHD iceberg. We are so much more than stereotypical neurodivergent traits.

To help you get to know yourself, we are going to dive deep below the surface of the ADHD iceberg in the Steps that follow. I am going to help you:

**Befriend the parts that make you:** your beginnings, early nurture, the place you began in society, and your current life circumstances.
**See your stories of joy and struggles for what they are:** they are the events that led you here. You did your best with the knowledge that you had at the time – and some of it was really good.
**Reframe your past experiences:** some of your struggles and joys shape your reality but they may also be a collective shared experience with others. Learn to approach your experiences with empathy, compassion and respect.
**Heal in safety:** don't try to do this work alone. Stick with those who empower you and show you compassion, rather than those who let their preconceived judgements remind you of the ways you need fixing. Work with a safe person (preferably a trained professional who understands your experience) who can stay present with you in your struggles until you can look at anything that triggers you through a new lens in the present moment, neither letting your past overcome you, nor letting it control your present interactions with others.

## Your Way Forward

When you learn more about who you are, you can begin the process of:

**Authenticity:** being true to your way of being, values, spirit and beliefs, even when it's difficult to do so. Your values, beliefs and actions are aligned. You take responsibility for your mistakes.

**Radical acceptance:** notice the parts that influence how you show up in daily interactions and navigate life's challenges and accept that some of these are younger parts of you, which caused you to derail in your life. Show them love.

**Self-forgiveness and self-compassion:** show yourself the kindness you deserve, and remember when you've acted out of fear. Allow space for the regret to surface. Perhaps you'd not been shown the appropriate way. Forgive yourself for your past behaviours.

**Repair, recovery and healing:** reach out to others to repair the rupture. If you were the one who was hurt, practise letting go of any disempowering narrative of victimhood that surfaces each time you feel alone. You are not alone. Form a coherent community with others and heal as part of a group.

**Thriving:** build the skills to create a happy life.

I'm going to be giving you guidance on all this and more in the chapters to come. But make no mistake. You will hit some bumps along the way. Please know that the journey on which we're about to embark will in no way mark the finality of your story. It is simply a transitionary period in your life.

You may still struggle to accept parts of yourself and at times allow preconceived notions and judgements to take over, such as accepting the medical model of psychiatry that leads us to believe we are broken. You may reject the parts of yourself that are wounded. It is precisely this separation from the self that makes us feel like we're not in the driver's seat of our lives, keeping us stuck in despair. If and when that happens, pour more love back into yourself. Keep focusing on centring yourself in your recovery, repair and healing through reframing your experience based on context and showing yourself compassion.

When we haven't learned to show ourselves compassion or love, we outsource that task to others. We risk constantly looking outside of ourselves for strength, inspiration, validation and love, so any contentment we experience may be fleeting, returning us to a state of discontentment when these people, events and things can no longer offer us what we need.

It's time to take back the power to run your life. To learn how to create a sense of safety within yourself. To regain control and drive your own recovery to become the boldest, brightest and most authentic manifestation of yourself.

Are you ready to go beneath the surface and gain a compassionate insight into what your label (or labels) means to you based on your reality? Part of this journey may lead you straight into the internal chaos you've been trying to avoid. Yet I urge you to embrace it. I will take you through a step-by-step process to excavate the layers that make you and rebuild your positivity so you can be the hero(ine) of your journey. And this is *your* story.

I know it's probably felt like a while since you were on the centre stage of your life, so I will help you reframe your neurodiverse experience via contexts that support your growth, to free you from the walls you built around your mind that have kept you from fully living the glorious life of your dreams.

Let's get started.

# Step 2: Expect to Discover Co-occurring Conditions

In 2020, before I was diagnosed with ADHD and autism, I was invited to speak about ADHD on LinkedIn Live, where over a thousand people showed up to listen to what I had to say. I can't tell you how that made me feel, but the following might give you an idea.

I'd already done extensive research and condensed my talking points to around eight to ten pages before the hour-long interview. When it came to it, I didn't even look at my notes. I was immersed in a state of flow because my research had become etched into my mind. I'd lived and breathed it. When my interviewer saw the level of research I'd done, she said, 'Oh my goodness Sam, are you doing a PhD in ADHD?'

There I was, having studied every article I could get my hands on, having listened to hundreds of podcasts, and having even created a social media campaign to ask the burning questions that were occupying my thoughts, doing it the way I'd always done. Today, I know this approach is called 'bottom-up thinking' and is often associated with the autistic learning and processing style, where we hoover up all the information we need so we have the necessary details to form our own conclusions eventually about something.[1] But it took me a further few months before I understood the significance of this.

Then, one day, someone in a community chat group shared how they were surprised to be called 'blunt' and how they had hurt other people's feelings without meaning to. I exclaimed, 'Oh, I've been told this too'. And another penny dropped. I looked up autistic traits on the internet. Now my jaw dropped:

- Special interests, check.
- Despising small talk, check.
- Having difficulty working out other people's intentions, check.
- Process thinking, check.
- Being unable to split your attention and attempts to do so often lead to sensory overwhelm, check (I guess?).

It wasn't until I spoke to my ADHD coach and she said, 'If you experience sensory sensitivities across multiple sensory systems, like touch, sound, light or body awareness, it could be a sign of neurodivergence, such as autism on top of ADHD. It's worth exploring further with a qualified professional.', that it made sense.

Cue flashbacks to all the times in my life when I've been called 'robotic', 'literal', 'blunt', 'serious', 'inflexible', 'controlling', 'unaware of seniority' and 'slow on the uptake'. This was in addition to contradictory traits like 'silly', 'fun', 'spontaneous', 'wild', 'free spirit' and 'likeable'. The uncanny thing is, these set of traits weren't always expressed consistently in my life. And this confused the people around me to the extent that my ex-husband once called me 'Jekyll and Hyde'.

Through comparing notes with others on how we showed up in the ADHD Girls community, it led me to the realization that it was more than ADHD we were dealing with. When you're diagnosed with ADHD, there is strong likelihood that you will have a co-occurring condition such as autism spectrum disorder (ASD). This awareness is the second stage of exploring the ADHD iceberg, because conditions such as ADHD and autism rarely appear in isolation.

So what exactly is ADHD when it co-occurs with ASD, and why does the latter frequently travel with ADHD? And what other neurodevelopmental/mental health conditions are we likely to unearth on this journey? Why are they known as comorbidities? (As we will come to see, this term often used to describe co-occurring conditions is itself flawed.)

Importantly, what happens when we consider the compounding impacts of living with multiple co-occurring conditions in society?

## THE LIMITATIONS OF LABELS

As we explored in Step 1, while once viewed primarily as a childhood behavioural issue largely focused on hyperactivity, impulsivity and distractibility, ADHD is now understood as a complex interplay of executive function, emotional regulation and attention differences – shaped by context, identity and environment. Despite expanded diagnostic criteria, the label still simplifies a deeply varied experience, especially as recent research shows that ADHD also encompasses a whole-body system experience. And much the same thing applies for ASD, which covers a broad continuum of traits loosely characterized as comprising deficits in social communication and interaction and repetitive behaviours, interests and activities. This is where it becomes a problem.

The ASD label attempts to capture a wide range of experiences, ranging from those who are considered 'high functioning' to those who require substantial support. But the clinical threshold for this often lacks objectivity and is largely based on a male standard, leading to many autistic females and other intersectional identities falling below the radar. Many autistic individuals who appear to function well externally may still struggle profoundly, often invisibly.

Emerging neuroscience, including recent insights shared by Gina Rippon, Professor Emeritus of Cognitive Neuroimaging, in *New Scientist*, challenges long-standing male-centric models of autism.[2] Studies are revealing that autistic girls often show *higher than expected social motivation*, with brain activity in areas related to social reward and social monitoring exceeding even that of neurotypical girls. Autistic girls also display *greater connectivity between social brain networks* and are more likely to suppress sensory over-responsiveness to avoid social embarrassment – pointing to a strong drive for social acceptance. These findings diverge sharply from traditional views of autism as marked by social aloofness or indifference.

What we're seeing instead is a pattern of camouflaging or masking: a conscious or unconscious effort to study, mimic and rehearse neurotypical social behaviours. This includes scripting interactions, eye contact and humour, often at great personal cost. Camouflaging is increasingly linked to chronic stress, anxiety and burnout, particularly in women and girls whose experiences have long been misread or overlooked by the existing diagnostic tools. These findings underscore the need to move beyond outdated stereotypes and broaden our understanding of autism and ADHD as they present across genders – and across lifetimes.

Given that the evidence suggests that ADHD and ASD have a co-occurring prevalence as high as 70–80 per cent in the UK population, this gives rise to further questions.[3] How we can neatly package traits under each of them, for example, when there are so many shared characteristics between these two conditions?

### THE RISE OF AUDHD: WHAT'S HAPPENING?

Professor Geraldine Dawson, Professor of Psychiatry and Behavioural Sciences and Director of the Duke Center for Autism and Brain Development, sums up the dilemma when she asks, 'Are we looking at one condition that's on a continuum, or two distinct conditions?'[4] As 30–80 per cent of autistic kids meet the criteria for ADHD and 20–50 per cent of kids with ADHD for ASD, researchers are now beginning to rethink the relationship between these two neurodevelopmental conditions.[5]

In fact, in AuDHD (the unofficial but popular term for co-occurring ADHD and ASD) the traits are often said to 'overlap'.

In 2016, in response to acknowledgement by the *Diagnostic and Statistical Manual of Mental Disorders* (DSM-5) that ASD and ADHD can co-occur, researchers became curious about the neurobiology and brain circuitry of AuDHD.[6] They looked at brain imaging of those with either ADHD or ASD, or both (AuDHD), and found that there are both shared and distinct brain features. ASD and ADHD have recognizably different and overlapping features in four key areas of brain function: paying attention, monitoring performance, recognizing faces, and processing sensory information.

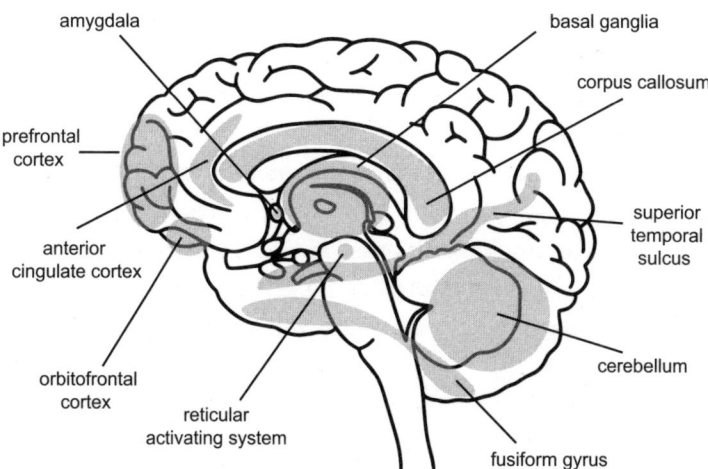

This diagram shows brain areas often linked to ADHD and ASD, such as the prefrontal cortex, amygdala, and cerebellum. But scientists now know that these conditions are not just about individual brain parts – they involve how whole brain networks communicate. In ADHD, this affects focus, emotional control and switching attention.[7]

In autism, it involves how people process social cues, sensory information and self-awareness. These brain differences happen across wide, connected systems, helping explain why symptoms can vary so much from person to person.[8]

ASD has been associated with affecting the following regions of the brain (however, these differences may present differently across sexes):

- The orbitofrontal cortex: May be underactive, making it harder to regulate emotions and navigate social norms. Linked to rigidity or literal thinking (social brain network).
- The superior temporal sulcus: Structural and functional differences here may lead to challenges interpreting social cues like facial expressions, voice tone or non-verbal cues (social brain network).
- The fusiform gyrus: May be less responsive, affecting facial recognition and emotional reading (social brain network).
- The amygdala: Often enlarged in autistic individuals, which may contribute to their increased fear or anxiety responses, particularly in social situations (salience and social brain networks), leading to heightened emotional reactivity, difficulty feeling safe in social environments, and a tendency to interpret ambiguous cues as threatening.
- The medial prefrontal cortex: atypical connectivity, supports theory of mind or understanding others' thoughts, leading to difficulty with perspective-taking (part of default mode and social brain networks).
- The cerebellum: Atypical size or connectivity, which may affect motor coordination and cognitive flexibility (part of broader attentional and motor networks).
- The corpus callosum: Often shows reduced volume or connectivity, which may contribute to slower or less integrated cognitive and emotional processing.

Meanwhile, in ADHD, the brain regions that are known to be affected are:

- The prefrontal cortex: Often shows reduced activity, affecting focus, planning and impulse control (central executive network).

## STEP 2: EXPECT TO DISCOVER CO-OCCURRING CONDITIONS

- The basal ganglia: Disruption here can interfere with motivation, reward sensitivity and habit formation (motor and executive networks).
- The amygdala: The amygdala is often reported to be smaller in ADHDers, but functionally hyperactive or overactivated in emotionally charged or frustrating situations, and is linked to impulsivity, frustration and emotional reactivity (salience and social brain networks).
- The anterior cingulate cortex: Irregular activation and plays a role in error detection, emotional regulation and task switching.
- The reticular activating system: Underactivity may cause difficulties with staying alert and sustaining attention (arousal and salience networks).
- The cerebellum: Can contribute to motor restlessness and problems with regulating attention (motor and attentional networks).
- The corpus callosum: Thinner or less connected in some cases, which may contribute to reduced cognitive integration and slower response inhibition.

In general, in one or both conditions, there is less robust wiring in the corpus callosum and in the cerebellum. As previously stated, amygdala size tends to be bigger in autistic people, but smaller in ADHDers. Total brain volume has been said to be bigger in autists than ADHDers too. What, then, happens when we possess both ASD and ADHD traits?

It turns out that AuDHD isn't autism *plus* ADHD, it's an entirely different neurotype.[9] A 2023 study has shown that the AuDHD brain has different brain dynamics compared to those of either ADHD or autism alone.[10] It seems that AuDHDers possess a blend of autistic socio-communication patterns but differ from pure ADHD in terms of their ADHD-like traits. AuDHD's 'ADHD', or its 'cognitive instability' trait, appears to arise in brain areas linked to flexible thinking and focus, rather than ADHD's attention and motor control. In 2023, a large, multi-site study of 75,000 people found evidence that there are distinct differences in ASD, ADHD and AuDHD brain anatomy. Perhaps more interestingly, they found what I'd always suspected: that the autistic brain differs anatomically by gender, and the ADHD brain differs by age.[11]

## ADDRESSING INDIVIDUAL NEEDS RATHER THAN LABELS

I will admit now that having read hundreds of research papers on ADHD, ASD, Tourette syndrome (TS), dyslexia, dyspraxia and mental health conditions in order to write this chapter, I feel browbeaten by the terminology that's often used. The words 'disorder' and 'impairment' are ubiquitous in medicine – if you've ADHD or are autistic, here's how you're impaired and need to be fixed. I'm not alone in thinking this is very patronizing.

Similarly, when describing co-occurring conditions, the term 'comorbidities' is sometimes still used. I haven't met a single neurodivergent who loves the word 'comorbidities', as it makes it impossible to avoid a doom-and-gloom outlook on ADHD and other co-occurring conditions.

Here are some neuro-affirming reasons why a word like 'comorbidities' should be retired:

**Outdated language:** the word 'comorbidities' was used pre-2013 to describe ADHD and other co-occurring conditions that were viewed as distinct diagnoses and that didn't go away even after ADHD is treated. Let's not forget that pre-2013, the criteria were tight, which meant only those who showed significant impairment would qualify for a diagnosis. AuDHD simply didn't exist in the eyes of the psychiatric community.

**Flaw in the label:** as we will see, we can take a 'dimensions' approach to neurodivergence traits, rather than labels, which will help us to understand that some of our traits manifest because our environment calls for them to be expressed, so they may fade away when we create more conducive environments for us to thrive, while enhancing our own resilience and skills to manage our neurodivergence.

**Situational understanding of mental health conditions:** as we understand the connection between biology, neurology and psychology (for example, the hormonal fluctuations in biological females in puberty, pregnancy, menopause), it becomes increasingly clear that some of the co-occurring conditions are situational, and mental health conditions such as generalized anxiety disorder (GAD), bipolar and major depressive disorder (MDD) can ebb and flow according to our life circumstances, and the people and events that happen within it. However, I draw the line when it comes to using neurodivergence and mental health conditions to justify potentially harmful or upsetting behaviours, and never as an excuse for them, especially if we end up causing harm to others.

**Negative language invites stigma:** the negativity surrounding the word comorbidities isn't helpful to the ADHD community, who may have an increased tendency for negative overthinking anyway. On the other side, it also creates a stigma in the eyes of the uninitiated – the world that the neurodivergents interact with. Instead, it's high time we started smashing misconceptions and explaining the neuro-affirming reasons behind observable behaviours.

There needs to be a shift towards empowering each of us to take back the power to run our lives. It begins with the words used to describe our experiences and it carries on in the stories we share with each other.

## BE EMPOWERED BY YOUR STORY

As the nuances of our neurodiverse experiences become more evident, psychiatrists will be placed increasingly under pressure to view each individual via the lens of their gender and life circumstances, as we will see in Step 4. When the power of identification and diagnosis lies largely in the hands of medical professionals, we need to be sure that the person in front of us is trained to understand how our neurodiverse experiences manifest themselves and to ask the questions that can uncover our unique hidden stories.

This is why before you even get to your assessment, you need to become empowered with all the knowledge you can acquire about yourself. However, this isn't always straightforward, given that some of us may struggle to understand the greater significance, or much less remember, what's happened in our own history. We may also have a biased view of the world based on our negative experiences and accord these more significance than the positive moments in our lives.

The seventh edition of the Publication Manual of the American Psychological Association paraphrased Social Comparison Theory, stating that in order to understand ourselves objectively, we need to be able to evaluate ourselves in comparison to others and then modify our behaviours and beliefs as necessary.[12] This may sound like a simple task, yet some autistic individuals can struggle to understand the emotional experiences of others when trying to make sense of how to act in social relationships. People with ASD traits can often wonder what other people's intentions really are or whether they're sincere, because many of us tend to accept things at face value and then we have to learn the hard way that people don't always mean what they say – that just because someone says that something is so, this doesn't necessarily mean it is so. In psychology and neuroscience, they call this the Theory of Mind deficit.

Similarly, for ADHDers, cognitive neuroscience has highlighted one of the challenges with executive function that is primarily regulated by our frontal lobes – metacognition, or thinking about our thinking, which means an awareness of your own thought processes that can create self-awareness. And if we do struggle with this, then surely the way that a neurodivergence assessment is currently set up is ableist at its core? For example, when you're at an assessment, there's a chance you may struggle to come up with the right words to describe a past situation, or you may have trouble recalling it exactly as it transpired, or, as one woman I know did, perhaps have no words (alexithymia) or the wrong words (dyslexithymia) to describe the feelings and thoughts relating to that event.

This is where sharing our stories really comes into its own. Due to the way we are wired as neurodivergents, we are more likely to derive the meaning from stories that invoke an emotional response within us. When I speak at ADHD and AuDHD women's community events, for example, women often tell me afterwards how sharing my story with so much vulnerability helped them find parallels in their own, making them feel seen and validated, and enabling them to move forward with healing – sometimes after holding on to pain and grudges for decades! Listening to another's courageous story can empower us to understand ourselves better, which in turn may give us the confidence to challenge an assessment outcome that we feel is unjustified.

## CO-OCCURRING CONDITIONS AS THE NORM, RATHER THAN THE EXCEPTION

You may already know, just as I do, that the joy of discovery of your neurotype doesn't end there. When you get diagnosed with ADHD or ASD later in life, there's a high chance you've been living with depression or anxiety, and perhaps other mental health challenges.[13]

Emeritus Professor Amanda Kirby, who has an international reputation in the field of neurodiversity, has been telling people for decades that we all have spiky profiles. Our neurodivergent traits may be expressed on a continuum from one label into another, rather than leaning dominantly towards one or the other. And even within the same label, there is diversity in how we show our neurodivergent traits. For example, if you get diagnosed with ADHD and identify with autistic, dyslexic or dyspraxic traits but don't express these via conventional stereotypes (as defined by DSM-5 and ICD-11, for example), then you may not meet the clinical threshold to receive these diagnoses. But it doesn't mean that you don't have the challenges.

The table below gives you an idea of some of the co-occurring neurodivergence, mental and physical health conditions that can accompany ADHD and autism. If any of these conditions ring any bells with you, don't panic, but start doing your own research. Knowledge is power and once you're aware of a potential problem, you can start to take steps to tackle it if necessary, such as getting the professional medical support you need. And of course you may find that none of the following applies to you at all, as everybody's different.

A Swedish study found that individuals with ADHD also have an increased susceptibility to chronic physical health conditions such as alcohol-related liver disease, sleep disorders, chronic obstructive pulmonary disease (COPD), epilepsy, fatty liver disease, obesity, cardiovascular disease, Parkinson's disease and dementia.[14] This list is by no means exhaustive, but it has certainly piqued my curiosity. Why do our neurodivergent traits tend to manifest not just in the brain but also in our bodies? What mechanisms are at play?

And what determines how and indeed whether these co-occurring conditions interact and show up for you in your daily life? Firstly, what does it look like in a child and an adult?

## STEP 2: EXPECT TO DISCOVER CO-OCCURRING CONDITIONS

| NEURODE-VELOPMENTAL/ MENTAL HEALTH CONDITION | PERCENTAGE OF THOSE WITH THE CONDITION ALSO SHOWING: |
|---|---|
| Tourette Syndrome (TS) | TS + ADHD: 35–90 per cent[15]<br>TS + ASD: 20 per cent[16] |
| Dyslexia | Dyslexia + ADHD: 25–40 per cent[17]<br>Dyslexia + ASD: up to 50 per cent[18] |
| Dyspraxia | Dyspraxia + ADHD: 50–89 per cent[19]<br>Dyspraxia + ASD: up to 50 per cent[20] |
| Dyscalculia | Dyscalculia + ADHD: up to 11 per cent[21]<br>Dyscalculia + ASD: 17–70 per cent[22] |
| Major Depressive Disorder (MDD) or Depression | MDD + ADHD: 30–68 per cent[23]<br>MDD + ASD: 40 per cent[24]<br>MDD + AuDHD: 40 per cent[25] |
| Generalized Anxiety Disorder (GAD) | GAD + ADHD: 50 per cent[26]<br>GAD + ASD: 50 per cent[27]<br>GAD + AuDHD: 69–72 per cent[28] |
| Substance Use Disorder (SUD) | SUD + ADHD: 15 per cent[29] |
| Sleep Disorder | ADHD + Sleep Disorder: 7.5 per cent had a sleep disorder diagnosis and 47.5 per cent had been prescribed sleep medication[30] |
| Obsessive Compulsive Disorder (OCD) | OCD + ADHD + ASD: up to 60 per cent[31] |

## Co-occurring Mental Health Conditions and Behavioural Patterns

Alexithymia
Anorexia nervosa
Binge eating disorder
Bipolar disorder
Complex post-traumatic stress disorder (CPTSD)
Conduct disorder
Dyslexithymia
Mood disorder
Obsessive-compulsive personality disorder (OCPD)
Oppositional defiant disorder (ODD)
Pathological demand avoidance (PDA)
Personality disorders
Post-traumatic stress disorder (PTSD)
Rejection sensitive dysphoria (RSD)
Schizophrenia[32,33]

## Co-occurring Physical Health Conditions

Adrenal fatigue
Asthma
Auditory processing disorder (APD)
Chronic fatigue syndrome (CFS)
Chronic pain
Delayed sleep phase syndrome
Diabetes
Eczema
Ehlers-Danlos syndrome (EDS)
Endometriosis
Fibromyalgia
Hashimoto's syndrome

> Heart disease
> Hypermobility
> Irlen's syndrome
> Irritable bowel syndrome
> Mast cell activation syndrome (MCAS)
> Migraine
> Pre-menstrual dysphoric disorder (PMDD)
> Postural orthostatic tachycardia syndrome (PoTS)
> Polycystic ovaries syndrome (PCOS)

## HOW DO THESE CONDITIONS INTERACT WITH ADHD?

Professor Peter Hill, who specializes in child and adolescent psychiatry, states that the way ADHD manifests changes as children mature through adolescence into adulthood:

> 'The problems you get with dyslexia, dyscalculia and Tourette tend to melt away as children mature into adults. In adults, you get high rates of anxiety, depression, substance use disorder and sleep problems. ADHD can be visualized as a vulnerability factor, where you can suffer from another condition that adds to the impairment, and this has a very important implication to assessment. There is up to 80 per cent chance of ADHD presenting with another condition that can magnify the disability or hide it.'[34]

It may be interesting to see how these types of neurodivergence tend to interact with each other, beginning in childhood.

### ADHD + ASD

Special interests, have specific ways of doing things and will be upset if parents or teachers do things in an unexpected way. Likely to consciously or unconsciously hide their natural behaviours and challenges to fit in or avoid judgement in nursery or school if they are able to. May experience separation and school anxiety until they have a nurturing adult or caring friends and feel like they are welcomed. Prone to show impulsive, disruptive and hyperactive traits. May not respond when called due to challenges in processing verbal and social cues. May have sensory sensitivities with school lunches, friendships and responding to instructions.

### AuDHD + APD

May or may not be hyperactive, may be able to hide difficulties if they are intelligent, sporty, or have 'roles' to play in school. Chatty and make friends easily, perhaps have challenges playing in a group and better at 1 to 1 interaction. Later in teenagehood, may be better able to hide their differences in a group. May not respond to name when called, may struggle to hear what a teacher is saying in a big class, challenges with processing verbal and social cues, which then affect language skills or lagging behind in certain subjects in school.

### AuDHD + APD + Dyspraxia

As above, with the added gross and fine motor skills challenges characteristic of dyspraxia, which may manifest as a delay in acquiring writing skills, using utensils to eat, buttoning clothes, tying shoelaces or braiding hair, being clumsy, falling, inaccuracy in gauging the distance between objects, challenges in hand-eye coordination, vertigo or dizziness.

### ADHD + Dyslexia

Common challenges in focus, information processing, working memory, finding the right words to describe their thoughts in an orderly sequence. Creative, out-of-box thinkers, innovative.

You might be wondering if there is anything in particular that contributes to these characteristic behaviours. One potential contributing factor could be the central unifying trait for all common forms of neurodivergence, and concerns challenges with our executive function, a set of mental processes that helps us carry out life tasks, set goals and implement them. Executive function is mediated by the prefrontal cortex, the part of the brain that matures later in adulthood. ADHDers can experience a neurodevelopmental delay in their prefrontal cortex by three to five years compared to their peers without ADHD. This affects our ability to carry out day-to-day tasks like planning and prioritizing, time management, working memory, organization, impulse control, task initiation, self-monitoring and self-regulation, flexible thinking, and attention and focus, which affects learning, processing information, and behaviour in school, home and social relationships.

## HOW DO CO-OCCURRING CONDITIONS AFFECT THE TRAJECTORY OF OUR LIVES?

As neurodivergent kids with multiple co-occurring conditions, we may go through the school system, friendship groups and our home life constantly needing to readjust our behaviours to fit in. The adaptation that is needed often comes at a cost to our self-esteem and mental health.

Then, as adults, our circumstances change – we are usually expected to become more independent, and our greatest challenges may shift from the executive function obstacles that prevented us from fitting in at school, to adapting to life in society, which requires adult skills such as communication, negotiating our personal needs, social and self-care skills. Sometimes, life throws a curve ball and we may find ourselves unable to cope when the demands become overwhelming. While we may have learned the skills that are needed to cope with one stage of life, the transition into the unknown may activate a pre-conditioned stress response. If left unsupported, this could even bring about mental and emotional health challenges.[35]

Researchers and clinicians are beginning to adopt a dimensional approach or focus on 'traits', rather than trying to connect genetics or neuroscience with diagnoses, as our behaviours can be inconsistent and mental health challenges like those just mentioned can ebb and flow throughout our lives.[36,37] However, the flipside is that overlapping traits can complicate diagnosis and treatment. The current guidelines recommend that when ADHD co-occurs with other conditions in adulthood, the most significant condition has to be addressed first.

It is important to emphasize that some of the behavioural traits we associate with conventional symptoms aren't fixed. Some of our coping strategies likely stem from adjusting to what our environment has demanded from us, and have since become a part of us, so it's more likely that we will notice new emerging traits as a result of our brain adaptations as we mature. That is not always the worst-case scenario, either.

When medical and psychiatric journals focus on 'impairment' when discussing neurodiversity, they neglect to see the foundation of our humanity, when one trait may very well compensate for the intensity of expression of another trait and can in some cases cancel out the perceived 'impairment'. At least until other changes come along to disrupt our ability to cope.

## PROCESSING THE DIFFERENT ASPECTS OF OUR IDENTITY

So how are we to go about processing our identity when it seems impossible to separate what is the result of nature from what is the result of nurture in our behaviours, or when the traits of our co-occurring conditions appear to contradict each other?

The experts and neurodiverse community don't always see eye to eye, but we unanimously agree on one thing – that there is so much diversity in our neurodiverse experiences that it's tough to get to the bottom of what's what. When you meet someone with a particular form of neurodivergence, you've met just the one person, not a stereotypical example of the condition.

And this is where the challenges lie. Medical and mental health professionals have typically diagnosed and misdiagnosed individuals based on behaviours that they can observe on the surface, drawing conclusions based on the best practice guidelines and what they themselves know at the time of assessment.

So what else might lie underneath these observable behaviours? How can we dig deeper in this second stage of our exploration of the ADHD iceberg?

In the table below, I bust some myths by presenting plausible reasons driving certain behaviours in the neurodiverse community, and how dealing with co-occurring conditions may change the ways that various aspects of AuDHD in particular interact with each other. Remember, our neurodivergence is situationally variable, which means our life circumstances can greatly influence how we behave.

Depending on our life stage, it's likely that we may see a dominant expression of one set of neurodivergence traits over another. Other factors that affect our behaviour, and which can contribute to our traits manifesting via a spectrum rather than 'all or nothing', are:

- Executive functioning differences
- Co-occurring conditions
- Coping strategies and adaptations, which include self-medicating behaviours
- Our physiological states, for example how well we've slept, eaten, rested, played which affect our neurotransmitters and hormones
- Life circumstances

As our understanding improves about how our neurodivergent traits interact, we will become more empowered to understand our own individual states and better equipped to find what we need to support ourselves at all stages of our lives. Our neurodivergence and mental health traits aren't fixed and can ebb and flow throughout the day, weeks, months and years along with our circumstances.

## Myth-busting How the Different Aspects of AuDHD Interact

| ASD STEREOTYPE | ADHD STEREOTYPE | HOW DO THESE TWO NEURODIVERGENCES INTERACT? | MYTH BUSTING |
|---|---|---|---|
| Autistic individuals are socially withdrawn | ADHDers are party animals | They may look like they are up for socializing and may make plans ahead of time, but may later find themselves with low energy reserves on the day and dread the social event. Due to the unpredictable nature of their energy levels, which can fluctuate with their biological and mental states, they may have developed social anxiety and often need to self-medicate to ensure they can appear in a socially acceptable state. To compensate, they may try to manage expectations by setting a limit to their social interactions and having an excuse ready to leave the event. | Their biology, nervous system and mental states can greatly influence the way they present. This can vary from time of day (when they feel most productive, if they've had something that stimulates their nervous system or sleep quality) to time of month (sex hormones and neurotransmitters for AuDHD women). As they absorb more sensory cues and absorb the emotions of others as though these are their own, it's likely that they need more time to recharge their energy and withdraw from socializing. However, as an AuDHDer who may struggle with social anxiety but also have a tendency to be hypersocial or hyper-talkative at times, they may sometimes miss the co-regulation that can come from wonderful connection. They may withdraw socially as they process their journey post-diagnosis and start ADHD medication, when their autistic traits may intensify. |

| ASD STEREO-TYPE | ADHD STEREO-TYPE | HOW DO THESE TWO NEURO-DIVERGENCES INTERACT? | MYTH BUSTING |
|---|---|---|---|
| Autistic individuals do not show emotions, lack empathy | ADHDers are 'too much', 'too soon', 'too personal' | AuDHDers may be chatty, impulsive, unfocused, but also seem thoughtful and capable of caring in a deep way, but may not always be able to demonstrate their emotions in real time. This can look like contrasting personalities, where they could potentially be really outgoing and extroverted one minute, and then it all changes when they seemingly have had enough. | They may have a real interest in people and strike up a new friendship but then find it hard to maintain it. Misunderstandings may arise from their literal way of communicating, which can come across as blunt despite them appearing to be sociable. With their slow processing of verbal and social cues, for example when they hear others share their news, they may feel it in their bodies (via affective empathy) but may not be able to show their feelings in real time. They may still be processing a conversation a week, months or years later, wishing they showed more socially acceptable reactions and facial expressions at the time! Those in a relationship with them may think they have alexithymia (inability to communicate thoughts and feelings) and when they do attempt to verbalize them, they could struggle with dyslexithymia (using the wrong words to describe a feeling). |

*(Continued)*

| ASD STEREOTYPE | ADHD STEREOTYPE | HOW DO THESE TWO NEURODIVERGENCES INTERACT? | MYTH BUSTING |
|---|---|---|---|
| Autistic individuals may have a preference for things staying the same | ADHDers may be bored in the same environment, and seek new sensations | AuDHDers may display polarizing behaviours such as wanting to control the outcome of every situation but also have a tendency to seek new experiences, which may look like booking a holiday on a whim or going on a spending spree despite being usually careful with money. In social or romantic relationships, they may fix their attention on a new person, may lose interest as the novelty wears off, or may stay too long in a relationship for fear of leaving familiarity and not having someone who understands their needs in their life. | AuDHDers can be sensation seeking when they feel bored, but may experience distress when realizing that they are out of their familiar environment, when they may need to recover from sensory overload and racing thoughts once they experience an overwhelming need to cope in the new environment. In the context of social or romantic relationships, sensory integration challenges can manifest as sensory seeking or sensory avoidance, which may give off a 'hot and cold' vibe. The outward dual personalities may mask distinct underlying emotional processes, where there are opposing parts within oneself as a result of adopting a chameleon-like identity from masking, which girls and women are known to be better at doing. |

# STEP 2: EXPECT TO DISCOVER CO-OCCURRING CONDITIONS

| ASD STEREOTYPE | ADHD STEREOTYPE | HOW DO THESE TWO NEURO-DIVERGENCES INTERACT? | MYTH BUSTING |
|---|---|---|---|
| | | They may also begin to show demand avoidance when they no longer want to comply with expectations if their heart isn't in it. | These traits can at times be misdiagnosed as a personality disorder as they can struggle to communicate their feelings (alexithymia or dyslexithymia) in a relationship and appear inconsistent. |
| Autistic individuals have a need to understand their plans and what is expected of them ahead of time | ADHDers don't think about what is needed until they are 'in it' and try to 'wing it' | AuDHDers may have a deep need for control and needing to plan well ahead of time, and this can appear like inflexibility; or they may also appear too relaxed if they are used to relying on others to create plans for them. The former individual is more likely to have developed anticipatory anxiety, where they obsess about putting strategies in place for a future event that causes anxiety in the moment to circumnavigate potential challenges. | As kids, they began in the world with a developmental delay in their prefrontal cortex, possessing what is deemed a weak working memory, being prone to forgetting things in the short term, told they are always late, and other self-regulation challenges. Together with a potentially enhanced amygdala that may predispose them to anxiety traits; they have an obsessive-compulsive trait brewing. When you add other maladaptive coping strategies to this, they can easily find themselves in need of support for GAD or OCD. |

*(Continued)*

| ASD STEREOTYPE | ADHD STEREOTYPE | HOW DO THESE TWO NEURODIVERGENCES INTERACT? | MYTH BUSTING |
|---|---|---|---|
| Autistic individuals need familiarity and routine | ADHDers thrive on throwing themselves into a new situation | AuDHDers can be a mystery wrapped in an enigma to themselves. They may feel the need to stick to their comfy rituals and routines that make them feel safe, but may also feel bored or lonely when things get too samey. You get someone who can be discontent when they've spent too long in one situation or insecure in a new situation with no guarantee for safety. This may look like starting new ventures or switching jobs when they need to get mental stimulation, and leaving when the motivation tapers. | Each aspect of neurodivergence can manifest as a dimension. The need for familiarity and routine may be born out of inflexibility in thinking, but they may throw caution to the wind if there is a reward that is aligned with their intrinsic values at the end of that pursuit. Autistic individuals may be motivated by a social purpose, too, and are often driven by their values. However, flying under the radar may have led to some self-medicating behaviours that enhance some of their ADHD traits, contributing to the incessant chatter in their heads, which may also cause challenges in knowing what is right for them when it comes to making decisions. Cue existential anxiety that can go on for as long as they are stuck in analysis paralysis. A polarizing personality may appear, confusing others who think they may be bipolar or have borderline personality disorder. |

| ASD STEREO-TYPE | ADHD STEREO-TYPE | HOW DO THESE TWO NEURO-DIVERGENCES INTERACT? | MYTH BUSTING |
| --- | --- | --- | --- |
| Autistic individuals have a need to dive deep and wide into their subject of interest | ADHDers may flit from one area of interest to another, and are good at looking at the big picture | AuDHDers may focus on a project for as long as they can learn more about it or their interests are held. They may display bottom-up thinking approach, wanting to find out everything about the subject, and then formulate the big picture idea. They may also be able to remember small details and fit them in places that they see constitute a logical process. | In the context of work, they've an interest-based nervous system that is motivated by interests, challenge, novelty, urgency and passion. Unless they are intrinsically interested in something, they may experience a persistent pull away from the task at hand. Even if they are interested at times, they may need some help to get stuck in, especially if it involves a new task that they are switching gears for. Their ability to hold large amounts of information in their minds due to the reduced synaptic pruning in the frontal lobe can, within a moment of clarity, help them connect the dots and contribute to a new way of doing and thinking. AuDHDers can be self-directed and may get to the top of their field if they're able to persist on their paths. |

*(Continued)*

| ASD STEREO-TYPE | ADHD STEREO-TYPE | HOW DO THESE TWO NEURO-DIVERGENCES INTERACT? | MYTH BUSTING |
|---|---|---|---|
| Autistic individuals have trouble dividing or switching their attention | ADHDers have challenges in focusing their attention | AuDHDers can find it difficult to both focus and divide their attention. This may manifest as someone who appears distracted when they are faced with boring and menial tasks, but can then be sucked into a strong tunnel of attention which is hard to get out of. The focus is strong and if distracted or needing to channel to more than one focal point, may cause a cognitive and sensory overwhelm. | The default mode network (where spontaneous thoughts pop up in the head and cause the minds to wander) within the AuDHD brain is almost always switched on, alongside their task positive network (which gets activated when they pay attention).[38] However, once they are in a flow state, it can be tough to switch gears. When asked to multi-task between two people or events, the autistic monotropic mind, which is typically better able to focus on a single stream rather than multiple streams, can encounter trauma as it is required to do more than it cognitively can. A monotropic split can cause meltdown or shutdown, leading them to feel anxious over time when unexpected demands are piled on them, or conjure demand avoidance. |

| ASD STEREO-TYPE | ADHD STEREO-TYPE | HOW DO THESE TWO NEURO-DIVERGENCES INTERACT? | MYTH BUSTING |
| --- | --- | --- | --- |
| Autistic individuals who don't comply to requests may be described as having pathological demand avoidance (PDA) | ADHDers may be people-pleasers | AuDHDers with PDA may have a strong sense of autonomy, avoid demands and have an anxiety-related need for control, especially when the demands of others are thought to be unreasonable. This may cause distress, as they also don't want to offend others. They may have difficulties with social relationships due to fear of committing to what others want from them, if they don't fulfil their own authentic needs first. | Pathological demand avoidance (PDA), or what neurodivergent advocate Tomlin Wildings has reframed 'Pervasive Drive for Autonomy', is a common profile under the autism spectrum. PDAers have an anxiety-driven need for autonomy, likely born out of an innately unique nervous system profile that has encountered early stressful life experiences when they enter traumatic situations they are unprepared for. This primes the nervous system for a fight-flight-or-freeze response. PDAers are thought to have higher levels of social capabilities than most autistic individuals, even if this may be on-the-surface skills rather than those sufficient to develop deeper relationships. AuDHDers with PDA tend to have a stronger need for novelty, are fully autonomous, and may withdraw from emotional demands too. |

## DEVELOPING A SITUATIONAL UNDERSTANDING OF OURSELVES

'Survivorship bias.' This was a phrase I learned early on when advocating for the understanding of neurodiversity in the workplace. It was used by the ADHD community itself to acknowledge that among those who identify with the same label, there are those who struggle and those who seem to have survived and thrived, having gone to university, got a good job, created a family unit, and appear to live a picture-perfect life. In fact, in the comments section in one of my Instagram posts, someone even said they thought I was someone who 'had survived ADHD'.

It may seem like this to the outside world, but then social media offers a small snapshot of my life. While I urge us to reframe our neurodiverse experiences from a position of strength, especially when advocating for ourselves in our work and personal relationships, I am aware that we need to constantly rebalance working with our strengths and supporting our challenges, and create environments where our challenges – including those from co-occurring conditions – will hopefully fade to the background.

In his article 'ADHD is a Whole-Life Experience' in *ADDitude* magazine,[39] Dr William Dodson, a psychiatrist who works with adults with ADHD, made the following points about ADHD concerning how the current approach to neurodiversity fails to take into account the nuances of our lives:

**Incomplete criteria:** the DSM focuses solely on childhood behaviours, leaving out crucial aspects of ADHD's impact on life at all ages.
**Emotional dysregulation:** emotional regulation is a major challenge for individuals with ADHD, but it's not addressed adequately. Emotions can be hard to study and measure, and are often masked due to embarrassment.

- **Age-related gap:** the ADHD criteria haven't been validated for adults, leaving a gap in understanding how ADHD affects grown individuals.
- **Lifelong experience:** ADHD remains constant throughout life, but individuals change as they face evolving life challenges.
- **Gender considerations:** ADHD research has historically overlooked women, perpetuating a misconception that they don't experience ADHD.

The full picture of ADHD includes emotions, age-related considerations and gender diversity. It's not just about behaviour. It's also about emotions, life impact and millions of people's wellbeing.

## Drawing On My Own Experience

The medical community knows that our neurodivergent traits worsen during periods of transition. The following are times when I struggled (and when this was balanced by having accountability and supportive people in my life):

- When I hit puberty at the age of 11, I was showing a lot of impulsive and sensation-seeking traits that got me into a world of trouble with my mum.
- I nearly failed all my exams, until I made a pact with my maths teacher that if she passed me, I would work harder. I achieved 100 per cent in the next test.
- A nurturing biology teacher sparked my love for biology at the age of 16.
- My autistic way of thinking and living at home (where I was nourished with healthy food) got me through school, and opened doors to obtain a scholarship to a postgraduate degree in the UK.
- Upon my moving to the UK, my ADHD traits were expressed more, and I started self-medicating with alcohol while seeking

social connection in the student party circuit! My 'train wreck' years ensued, saved by the final push for my PhD.
- I entered the world of work and felt lost. A decade-long existential crisis ensued in which I job hopped (across 16 different industries to date), went inward, and became a mother. I experienced many mental health challenges in various transitions.
- I became a second-time mum and had postnatal anxiety, following notable changes in how my hormones were behaving.
- I got diagnosed with ADHD in the pandemic, and I identify as autistic too.
- I started ADHD medication and found it hard to take a break from work.
- A period of burnout ensued that I'm still recovering from.
- I received my autism assessment at the age of 43 – and AuDHD explains so much!

Having been someone who's experienced the 'high highs and low lows', I wanted to add a caveat to what Dr Dodson says in his article. I believe that rather than 'ADHD remains constant throughout life, but individuals change as they face evolving life challenges', it's more about the way circumstances and demands evolve throughout our lives that will invite the expression of certain traits within our neurotype. Whether these are, for example, ADHD, autistic, compulsive, depressive traits or not really depends on how we adapt to our unique situation, significant relationships, and the support we have in place.

### EQUIPPING YOURSELF WITH KNOWLEDGE

Apart from the brain differences that come with possessing co-occurring conditions, the following are some of the factors that can contribute to the nuances in the way we present due to the diversity of our experiences:

- Gender
- Cognitive ability
- Development across the lifespan
- Trauma from our beginnings and life in motion
- Large hormonal transitions (for biological women during puberty, pregnancy, perimenopause)
- Environmental triggers
- The quality of our social and personal relationships
- Coping and maladaptive mechanisms
- The presence of a supportive network
- Lifestyle
- Response to treatment
- Cultural considerations
- Hidden stories of social oppression (gender, race, social class, religion, migration and others)
- Life circumstances later in life

Being aware of these factors is crucial for a comprehensive understanding of our conditions and for tailoring holistic interventions that address our specific needs. There are those who succeeded because their life circumstances worked for them, whether through luck, support or interdependence. However, there are also those who succeeded at a cost to their mental health. And there are neurodivergents who struggled and needed substantial support before being able to thrive.

Then there are those who functioned until a large life or hormonal transition came at them. This is where our prior experiences of resilience determine our ability to cope. Professor Peter Hill has described ADHD as a 'vulnerability factor'[40], and while I don't want to paint us as vulnerable, I much prefer to think that, yes, we are sensitive to the world.

We are all born with a set of genes that will predispose us to certain personalities, diseases and sensitivities. Given that a selection of traits that is unique to your blood line is embedded within your genes, there are things you can change and things you can't. For example, outcome studies on personality showed that traits such as intelligence, aggression and alcoholism are passed down the family lineage, and the environment in which you grow up can influence the degree to which you manifest these traits for better or worse.[41] For these reasons and others, if you have ADHD and a spectrum of other co-occurring traits which can sensitize you to a range of physical and mental health conditions, surely the thing to do is to be aware of what those triggers and environments are, avoid them, and fill your life with habits and routines that protect you against the development of these conditions? In other words, you should create a physical and mental health disorder prevention programme for ADHD, or whatever your neurotype is.

You need to begin by taking stock of what traits or symptoms you are dealing with. What are your mental challenges? What are the physical challenges? How are these challenges affecting your daily life?

Coping strategies are adaptations and may have become so embedded into our day-to-day lives that we may not even know we rely on them, and they can include things like substance misuse, addiction to things, people or ways of doing things (see Step 4, page 134). Unfortunately, sometimes if our immediate environment doesn't favour the good and healthy, we may develop maladaptive strategies in the form of self-medicating behaviours. The cost of maladaptive habits can be an impact on our nervous system or stress response, causing abuse to self or others, trauma in our relationships, or unfulfilled potential.

If the strategies you use to help you get through the day have had a cost on your mental health and affect your ability to live a healthy and satisfying life, then you need to be prepared to change your habits and circumstances.

## How do You Interact with the Demands of the World Around You?

The following are prompts designed to help you understand whether your environment or circumstances work for you or not:

1. Can you cope with the demands of your day-to-day life? If so, are your coping strategies helpful?
2. Is there something within your environment that has bothered you, perhaps for longer than you want to admit?
3. Are there any changes in your context that affect your ability to cope, where you were once able to?
4. If your coping strategies are not helpful in the days or months after employing them, can you adopt healthier ways of coping? Is there anyone you can ask for help to start the ball rolling?
5. Are your environment and circumstances conducive for you to thrive?

**Reflection**
It can be helpful to keep a diary of your day-to-day habits, routines and behaviours to derive a picture of what is at play. Can you spot a pattern in terms of what actions help you achieve a state of balance versus what knocks you out of sync?

### TAKING BACK CONTROL

When neurodivergents live in a state of prolonged chronic stress and suffer from burnout, this can look like depression. So, when you try to get to the root of what led you there, where do you start?

As our current understanding around ADHD and autism changes, it's important to note where in your life you've significant needs that aren't being met, and to work on pulling in support in those areas. You can begin by exploring the hidden layers of the ADHD iceberg and by going beneath the surface of the behaviours to discover what you need. As Doctor Gabor Maté said in his book *The Myth of Normal*,[42] in his experience as a clinician, it is the 'patients' who ask all the questions to figure out their best way forward who have the best outcomes.

It is what we do with the hand we are given that makes all the difference.

## What Do You Need?

You can begin to devise a menu of your mental, physical, social and emotional needs, so that you can work out which circumstances help you to thrive. Here are some questions you can ask yourself that can lead to some revelation around what you can change:

**Mental needs**

1. Are you able to get engaged with something that interests you?
2. What ways do you best learn, process and retain information?
3. Is there a time of day when you feel especially productive?
4. What do you need to do your best work?

**Physical needs**

1. Is medication advised and is it something you would like to try?
2. Are there changes in your energy levels that need addressing?
3. Does your lifestyle support your health and wellbeing: nutrition, sleep, exercise, managing stress levels, hormonal health?

> 4. Are you aware of any life or hormonal transitions that can affect your health and wellbeing?
> 5. What demands are present in your life stage right now that potentially affect your ability to look after your health?
>
> **Social and emotional needs**
>
> 1. Do the social relationships you have nourish you and enhance your energy and creativity?
> 2. Do you carve out time to spend with people who matter most to you?
> 3. Are your loved ones understanding of who you are and what you want to achieve in life?
> 4. Do your personal relationships add value to your life?
> 5. Are you aware of your energy levels and able to take stock of when they are becoming depleted so you can recharge?
> 6. Do you have habits and routines that help you rebalance your nervous system?

The discussion about ADHD and co-occurring conditions becomes much more empowering when we revisit the language and the labels used around them and start to advocate for our neurodivergent strengths. It's important to understand how our co-occurring traits can be influenced by our circumstances and, empowered by our own stories, we can start removing the barriers so we can fulfil our potential.

Part of this journey is about learning how to show up better and authentically. It is important to note that we have a varying spectrum of needs and strengths, and it looks like our focus should therefore very much shift towards creating holistic strategies to support ourselves. These strategies need to be tailored to our individual needs, including where we've come from as well as where we want to go. Which takes us to the next layer of the ADHD iceberg, and understanding our nature.

# Step 3: Understand Your Nature

'My ADHD makes me appear like I'm disorganized and forgetful at times, but I'm able to focus when it's something I have an intense interest in.' When I speak to ADHDers, this is a line I hear a lot, but what's your ADHD like? And why is it very likely different to mine?

Within the community of late-diagnosed ADHDers, there is a sense of curiosity around the way our neurodivergence shows up and what causes the ADHD experience to be so diverse, yet have some shared similarities. Is it a case of nature or nurture, or perhaps both?

To begin to unpack this, we first need to know a bit about how the biology works – from the cellular level to the entire human being. That's why in this chapter, we're going to take a look at the genetic building blocks that we inherit from our parents, which help make us who we are, and we'll see how these can make us predisposed to various conditions and sensitivities. Once we're aware of these sensitivities, we can begin to take practical steps by adjusting daily choices around things like our diet to tackle them.

## MY OWN WAKE-UP CALL

I was diagnosed with ADHD just before I turned 40, shortly after I had my second child. It would be another eight months before I came around to the idea of starting a class 2 drug, first weaning my son off breastfeeding before I began taking lisdexamfetamine. Until then, I was only aware of the cognitive and mental health symptoms of ADHD, which I believed the medication was helping with as it increased the levels of the neurotransmitters dopamine and norepinephrine that are apparently reduced in the ADHD brain.

| PROS OF MY MEDICATION | CONS OF MY MEDICATION |
| --- | --- |
| Increased my confidence | Reduced my appetite after breakfast |
| Gave me mental focus and clarity for longer periods in the day | Made me forget to drink water |
| Made me feel content (at a dosage that feels just right for me) | Increased my already over-focused tendency when it was something I was interested in, making it harder for me to switch gears outside work |
|  | Interfered with my ability to switch off |
|  | Interfered with my ability to practise a good sleep hygiene and led to four years of less-than-ideal sleep quality |

While I was on the medication, my neurodivergence manifested as over-focusing on any problem I was trying to solve and in doing the same thing over and over again. As my business grew and demands for my speaking increased, I found it hard to juggle this with parenting and then co-parenting. My physical health symptoms increased, including:

- Anxiety and brain fog
- Fatigue and chronic stress
- Menstrual irregularities
- Mental and emotional burnout

- Mood swings
- Sensitivity to cold and heat
- Social anxiety
- Sleep troubles

All the while, I was fixated on the idea of oestrogen being an indirect regulator of dopamine, and how if my oestrogen levels fluctuated throughout the month, then my dopamine levels would too. This led to me adjusting my medication to two dosages, with 30mg in the first half of my cycle as my oestrogen levels increased in the lead up to ovulation, changing to 40mg when I entered luteal phase, being mindful of any potential changes in my moods. (I'll be talking about the influence of hormones in a little more detail in Step 4, but I am just mentioning it in passing here, as it turns out that it wasn't the only factor at play, as you'll see.)

Over time, my physical symptoms appeared to compound and have an effect on one another. I was in a state of chronic stress and overwhelm, I ate and slept poorly, and woke up with brain fog for most of that year.

And then something weird happened.

I went away on a yoga retreat.

I ate a glorious buffet of vegan food three times a day for three days. I did yoga round the clock. I fell asleep to soothing mantras and had seven to eight hours of sleep even if I was still tossing and turning. It was the ultimate stress reset.

Yes, I was still emotional, but I also felt calm and at peace. This was also during my luteal phase right before my period, when I was 'supposedly' going to have a more difficult time. When I got back from my yoga retreat, I did a blood test and my sex hormone levels were normal. I didn't struggle with the usual premenstrual symptoms. I was shocked.

A month later and a heap more work and life demands descended on me. In March, I was juggling 20 keynote speaking engagements with writing the first chapter of this book, alongside co-parenting two neurodivergent kids and maintaining a new relationship.

I kept trying to de-stress as I went. However, a lot of the frustration of my setup had nowhere to go . . . but right into my heart. My blood pressure went up to levels considered high for my age and gender, and I could feel intense heart palpitations, as though my heart was pumping more blood rigorously through my blood vessels, which made it difficult for me to breathe. My back muscles were strained and hurt. It was so painful I couldn't even stretch when I did yoga.

In the midst of giving a talk in a swanky office in Farringdon, I stopped breathing. I can confirm that it is possible to carry on talking as you catch your breath, because I did it. I continued to speak while not breathing for what felt like forever. I felt overwhelmed by emotional and sensory stress, and I found that I needed to press my hand on my heart so I could take each breath. My breathing was so unreliable that I couldn't walk for more than three metres without having a panic attack. I thought I was going to die. All the while, I was imagining how the stress hormone cortisol affected both oestrogen and dopamine, and how that then reduced the capacity of other bodily functions.

I knew the first thing I had to do was to reduce my stress, but where in the world should I start? Looking out into the audience at that International Women's Day event, I knew I had to recover.

I felt the weakest I had ever been. I could deal with the cognitive burnout I had from my work, but the sensory and emotional burnout from co-parenting while navigating divorce was harder to manage. I had also been in trauma therapy for over a year, trying to undo a lot of my unhealthy coping mechanisms. And I was reliving a lot of the pain from the past, without the tools to manage this in the present.

So, what brought me to that point? Why did I become so stressed that I thought I was on the point of complete collapse? At a fundamental level, it's because of the way that humans like us are made.

## ADHD AND YOUR FAMILY TREE

Let's start with the basics, although admittedly they're pretty miraculous as basics go: the DNA we inherit from our parents consists of genes that form segments which help determine our characteristics and traits. In this respect, you could compare our genes to the colours set out on an artist's palette. They show the potential, but they aren't the finished painting.

A significant part of the explanation of our neurodivergence manifestations comes from the genetic mutations we inherit from our parents. Researchers agree that ADHD can be passed down a family blood line, with some studies postulating that ADHD has heritability rates of 60–90 per cent.[1] However, there isn't one single gene that has been found to be responsible for this neurodivergence, but 76 genes and counting. It's a polygenic phenomenon, in which multiple genes interact to contribute to the appearance of traits that we see in ADHD, such as impulsivity, hyperactivity, inattention and emotional dysregulation. Underneath these observable traits, often there are myriad causes relating to sleep issues, energy production, neurotransmitter and hormonal regulation and stress response – down to a potential inability to break down caffeine and alcohol, which are examples of the fundamental biological mechanisms that underlie an ADHDer's day-to-day life.

Curiously, many of these genes contain mutations or natural variations (known as variants) that are commonly found in the human genome, with a subset being rarer forms of gene variants.

## FROM GENES TO METABOLIC PATHWAYS AND THE WHOLE SYSTEM

If you are an ADHDer or an AuDHDer, you've probably noticed that your challenges don't stop at the level of your focus, executive dysfunction or social struggles. Maybe you've also got chronic pain. Gut issues. Hormonal chaos. Fatigue that won't budge. Autoimmune conditions. Sleep issues. A nervous system that feels like it's always stuck in 'ON' or even 'OFF'. You're not imagining it – and you're definitely not alone. ADHD and autism are complex, multi-factorial conditions. They're not caused by one single gene or brain mechanism, but rather by a symphony of interacting factors, including how our genes influence the way our cells function across our entire body.

Research into ADHD has uncovered gene variants that impact neurotransmitter metabolism, energy production, inflammation, detoxification and methylation – all fundamental cellular processes. These effects aren't limited to your brain: many of the genes associated with ADHD are expressed in up to 54 different tissue types in the body – including your heart, liver, blood, reproductive organs, bones, muscles, gut, thyroid and even your skin.[2]

For example, genes like MAOA, MAOB, COMT and MTHFR don't just affect how your brain works – they also help regulate your stress response, hormone balance, detox capacity and inflammation levels. Gene variants can alter the typical process of using micro- and macronutrients such as B vitamins (B6, B12 and so on) and omega-3 fatty acids, and affect important metabolic functions. Genetic differences alter metabolites (the small molecules that fuel all the chemical reactions in your cells), which in turn affect everything from your energy cycles to immune function.

Take MTHFR as a well-known example. This gene affects your ability to convert folate (vitamin B9) into its active form, methylfolate, which is crucial for:

- Making serotonin and dopamine
- Reducing inflammation and homocysteine
- Supporting detoxification and antioxidant production
- Regulating gene expression (aka epigenetics – how your body turns genes 'on' and 'off')

When these processes are disrupted, the effects can ripple through your entire system, impacting your mental, physical and emotional health. For example, chronic fatigue and pain conditions such as fibromyalgia, hypermobility and endometriosis often show up alongside ADHD and autism. Your body might be struggling to produce enough cellular energy or manage inflammation because of underlying metabolic dysfunctions. At the genetic level, changes in the genes DRD4, SLC6A3 and MAOA affect how your brain processes dopamine and serotonin, influencing both pain levels and motivation. Some of the metabolic pathways that may be out of sync in these conditions may be mitochondrial dysfunction and inflammation, which interfere with energy production, leaving you with fatigue, brain fog and heightened pain sensitivity.

With regards to hormonal health of biological females, from premenstrual dysphoric disorder (PMDD) and polycystic ovary syndrome (PCOS) to perimenopause and endometriosis, hormonal issues often coexist with ADHD/autism. These aren't separate problems; they're often connected through shared metabolic pathways. This is why even when you start hormonal replacement therapy and expect your symptoms to get better, they may not so you need to look at gene variants such as COMT or NR3C1 which impact oestrogen clearance and hormone sensitivity, as well as metabolic pathways that can cause glucose imbalances, poor detox and chronic inflammation, disrupting hormone production and signalling. Hormonal imbalance isn't 'just hormones', it also involves our neurobiology and metabolism.

This is why I've said that diagnosis doesn't always equal support, as 'treating ADHD' often doesn't begin to touch the fatigue, gut issues or stress overload we experience. Understanding this can help you make sense of your symptoms (you're not lazy or broken), get more personalized care (beyond the standard ADHD medication), advocate for testing or supplements of micronutrients and macronutrients to support your body's actual needs, and understand how stress, inflammation and burnout affect you more deeply.

Maybe you've tried things like improving your sleep hygiene, using focus tools or meds, and you still feel drained. It could be because your cellular energy systems are struggling. Mitochondria (your energy-makers) are often underpowered in ADHD due to these genetic variants.

## THE BRAIN ENERGY THEORY

While researching metabolites implicated in ADHD, autism and other mental health conditions, I found many that are involved in cellular energy production and utilization by the mitochondria, the cell's powerhouse. A theory that emerged recently around the manifestation of symptoms of mental health conditions is the brain energy theory outlined by Harvard psychiatrist Dr Chris Palmer in his book *Brain Energy*.[3] This theory brings together all the schools of thought around the contributing causes of mitochondria function in the brain, such as metabolic impairments caused by genetics, epigenetics, hormonal changes, lifestyle factors like diet and nutrition, stress, inflammation and oxidative stress.

Without energy, a cell will struggle to perform its normal functions, that is to make new cells, make proteins, transport chemicals within the cell and from one cell to another, as well as getting rid of cells (or structures within it) that no longer work. When cells don't have enough energy to create proteins to facilitate biological pathways and elicit cellular functions, it may lead to malfunction of processes, rendering them either underactive, overactive, or not active at all, upsetting homeostasis – the body's ability to maintain inner stability in the face of external changing conditions.

The theory of brain energy makes a lot of sense, as it certainly helps us link what happens in our bodies with how it manifests in the mind. Researchers also believe that understanding the metabolic signatures of disease manifestations, the small metabolites detected in our biofluids, will bridge the gap between the genes we inherit and how we manifest our symptoms. From where I'm sitting, I think it could help to explain how you show up with ADHD in your day-to-day life, especially with your energy levels, what it could render you vulnerable to, and what you can do to help yourself.

## THE DEVELOPING ADHD BRAIN

We saw in Step 2 how researchers have found that in kids with ADHD, there is a notable delay of three to five years in the development of the prefrontal cortex, with reduced dopamine and norepinephrine signalling within the frontal lobe (the brain control centre that regulates day-to-day tasks such as reasoning and voluntary movements), the limbic system (the emotional brain), as well as between these parts, and the reticular activating system (which filters out unnecessary information so important stuff gets through to regulate behaviour and motivation).

This, alongside other co-occurring conditions such as dyspraxia, can impact the development of fine and gross motor skills. The former affects efficiency of early pencil grip, which manifests as quality of early or lifelong handwriting proficiency. The latter affects our coordination and balance. Add auditory processing differences to this and you get a picture of the challenges that may surface during somebody's life.

On a related note, a fantastic review looked at the timeline of the developing brain in predicting the risk of psychiatric conditions. According to its findings, neurodevelopmental conditions such as ADHD tend to show up early, before a child reaches the age of ten, while anxiety disorders, schizophrenia and substance abuse tend to show up between the ages of ten and twenty, with mood disorders occurring around age twenty-five.[4]

Here's what's potentially at play. A child's sensorimotor complex, which regulates their movements, tends to mature first. If they've got ADHD, this will tend to manifest first in childhood as having plenty of motor energy and drive before they've developed the brain-based brakes (otherwise known as impulse control and inhibitory function), and so they can show up as disruptive, hyperactive and impulsive.

Next up is the amygdala, which is the major processing centre for emotions and links our emotions to other brain functions such as memory, learning and sensory processing. The amygdala plays a pivotal role in one of our earliest and most primitive needs, the development of the brain circuitry for our threat response, which makes us feel fear and anxiety so we can mobilize and run from a threatening environment. Anxiety disorders tend to manifest in the cusp between childhood and adolescence, but in children with ADHD, this can manifest earlier due to neurodevelopmental differences in the following:

- Over-responsive amygdala (responsible for detecting threats, emotional processing and responses)
- Delayed maturation of prefrontal cortex (responsible for executive function, rational decision-making, and long-term goal-directed purpose)
- Under-responsive ventral striatum (induce reward- and sensation-seeking behaviours)

To paraphrase the words of neuroscientist Robert Sapolsky in his book *Determined*, adolescence is this wild in-between phase when dopamine is running the show, but the prefrontal cortex – the part of the brain that helps us think ahead, regulate emotions and make good decisions – is still under construction. It's actually the last part of the brain to fully develop, and interestingly, it's also the part that is shaped most by experience rather than genetics. That delay might exist for a reason, and our environment, relationships and the things we go through can help sculpt how we learn to navigate the world.

The dopamine system is usually going full steam by the time we're 11 or 12 years old, but in ADHDers, this may look more like a dysregulation of dopamine, norepinephrine and other neurotransmitters, which could lead to compensatory or extreme forms of behaviour in a bid to get stimulation; alternatively, it may manifest in a stronger emotional response to disappointment. The amygdala can behave differently in ADHD brains. If you haven't had the chance to learn how to understand, name and regulate your emotions – whether due to your environment, neurobiology or both – this can lead to emotional dysregulation. In other words, your emotional 'alarm system' might be firing too often, too intensely, or in ways that feel hard to control. Meanwhile, the prefrontal cortex is half-baked and in ADHDers, there is a further delay in the maturation of the frontal lobe compared to those without ADHD. The developmental imbalances between these brain structures in ADHDers means that we are going to have fewer tools and therefore less brain efficiency to make sense of the experiences we encounter by ourselves, so we may need more support from our caregivers.

### The Importance of Protecting Young Neurodivergents

As our brains are plastic, we are malleable by the sum of adverse childhood experiences (ACEs) and protective experiences that occur in our childhood through to early adolescence. It is so imperative that, as adults, we know this and can help the younger generation of neurodivergents because if they encounter early trauma without the support to understand what they are going through, it can change the developmental trajectory of their fear and anxiety systems. Research has shown that when a child's early environment lacks consistent emotional safety – whether due to stress, overwhelm or breakdowns in connection – it can shift the timing of prefrontal and cortical development, the most recently evolved part of the human brain.[5]

According to Robert Sapolsky, late adolescence and early adulthood are when your environment really starts shaping the kind of frontal cortex you'll have as an adult. Since the frontal cortex is the last brain region to fully mature, it's also the one most influenced by what you go through and how you experience the world – rather than being hardwired by your genes. And it makes sense that it works this way, right? The frontal cortex helps with those tricky, nuanced decisions like doing the right thing even when that's tough. It has to process all the grey areas – like knowing when it's okay to break the rules or navigating things like hypocrisy and self-interest – and there's no genetic map for that. It takes about 25 years for the frontal cortex to figure all of that out.

It doesn't help that in ADHDers, the prefrontal cortex doesn't reach full maturity until their mid-thirties or early forties, so if they're using this time to self-medicate in ways that negatively impact the health of their frontal cortex, then they are likely heading into adulthood collecting experiences that will render them underequipped to handle life's difficulties – perhaps leading to significant mental health challenges along the way. We are potentially looking at a child or teen who enters every class, school and the home environment primed with a nervous system that has sensed and felt too much. They've adapted to the stressors in everyday life with a survival response – fight, flee (avoid), freeze (dissociate), fawn, and/or fib. Over time, these responses risk becoming embedded in their neural pathways as repeating patterns of behaviour.

A 2023 study published in *Nature Medicine* looked into brain scans and found that adolescents with more symptoms of mental health conditions, autism or ADHD have undergone less pruning than usual of synaptic connections between neurons.[6] The researchers believe that the lack of pruning contributes to more 'white noise' within the frontal lobes. Study participants with this pruning defect also carried the gene IGSF11, which had previously been associated with multiple mental health disorders.

As our frontal cortex is the part of the brain most shaped by our experiences and environment, our upbringing will strongly colour the nuances of our neurodiverse experiences in adult life, too. However, as we will see in Step 4, while our personal circumstances help to shape the diverse ways in which ADHD manifests in our lives, at a fundamental level our genetic inheritance predisposes us as a collective to react to the world in certain ways.

### What an Adolescent with ADHD May Experience

- The inefficiency of delayed executive functioning, leading to delay or trouble in processing information, thoughts, feelings, controlling impulses and behaving appropriately in social situations.

- Masking to hide the differences.
- Imbalanced dopamine and norepinephrine levels, leading to compensatory behaviours.
- A nervous system primed to respond to particular environments and interactions with a hyperactivated stress response, unless they're supported.
- Less pruning in the neuronal synaptic connections in the frontal lobes, leading to less efficient brain circuitry and goal-directed long-term thinking.

## OUR COLLECTIVE EXPERIENCES

Given our genetic predispositions, you might be getting a slightly clearer picture of why many neurodivergents are at increased risk of experiencing chronic health conditions or complain of long-term physical ailments.

In Step 2, we considered how ADHD is associated with a wide range of co-occurring physical health conditions (see page 53), while earlier in this Step, I highlighted some of the gene variants and metabolic pathways implicated in neurodivergence and also how the brain develops differently in individuals with ADHD. When we zoom out and look at the organ systems where common physical health conditions occur in those with ADHD, we can see that they include the nervous, cardiovascular, respiratory and musculoskeletal systems, and metabolic diseases.

So why are ADHDers predominantly affected in the systems that relate to feeling, managing stress, burning energy, movement and breathing?

To begin to understand this, we need to look at the body and brain as an interconnected macrosystem, where individual systems are constantly interacting and striving for homeostasis to elicit healthy biological functions. Earlier I mentioned homeostasis, which is a self-regulating process in our bodies whereby biological systems work in sync to maintain stability in the face of external changing conditions. Read that again. Now think for a minute about what neurodivergents are dealing with when they find themselves constantly trying to navigate external changing conditions, when their internal conditions are often characterized by the apparent contradictions of chaos and inflexibility.

As a collective, neurodivergents share one thing in common: we have inherited an increased sensitivity to the world. This sensitivity isn't made up. The difficulties this creates aren't made up either. The trouble is, it's invisible. And because of this, our bodies are constantly working doubly hard to readjust to what life throws at them. This is why in an effort to feel better and cope with the expectations of others, we tend to pressure ourselves and self-medicate to enable us to have the energy to show up in our lives and fulfil demands that may exceed our ability to cope, and which push us to the point of no return. All of which brings me to one of my favourite subjects – our relationship with stress.

## STRESS

Stress is our physical and physiological response to stressors that challenge our normal functioning (maintained via homeostasis). It's a normal part of life, and a healthy dose of stress can be good for us: it boosts our memory, keeps us motivated, and helps us feel energized and performing at our best.

When we encounter a stressor, the amygdala (our brain's emotion processor) sends a signal to the hypothalamus, which communicates with the body through the autonomic nervous system (ANS) to elicit a stress response. The autonomic nervous system has two branches, the sympathetic nervous system (SNS) and parasympathetic nervous system (PNS). You can look at the sympathetic branch as a gas pedal, and the parasympathetic branch as the brake. When the former is activated, epinephrine (adrenaline) and sugar flood the bloodstream, and the fight-or-flight response is activated. This wiring is so efficient that the response happens before the brain has a chance to process what is happening. When adrenaline subsides, the hypothalamus then activates the second route of the stress response – the HPA (hypothalamus-pituitary-adrenal) axis, where hormone signals are sent to the adrenal glands to release cortisol, helping the body to stay primed for threat. When a stressor passes, the parasympathetic branch is activated, promoting the 'rest and digest' response to calm the body down.

Many neurodivergents have a complicated relationship with stress – while we may go in search of it to activate our brains, living with conditions such as ADHD and autism can itself produce stress. As touched upon earlier, in both of these types of neurodivergence, researchers have found gene variants that predispose us to challenges in regulating adrenaline, noradrenaline and dopamine homeostasis. These chemicals help control the body's reaction to stress, focus and energy levels, and they also play a role in feelings of reward and motivation. And so, the dysregulation in these chemicals can look like an atypical stress response, increased sensory sensitivities and imbalanced neurotransmitters.

If you think about it, the self-regulation challenges due to a delayed maturation of the prefrontal cortex, on top of our sensory integration challenges, makes ADHD a stress-producing condition in itself!

In our adult life, the difficulty in managing the levels of neurotransmitters can show up in our not being able to reliably regulate our behaviour and emotions, mood, impulse control, focus and communication.

It's not surprising that we have learned to adapt as neurodivergents through manifesting other behaviours in response to stress – the fight, flight, freeze, fawn and fib, which only serves to put us in a prolonged state of sympathetic activation. To understand our stress response, it's important to know that neurodivergents generally have what is called a 'rigid nervous system' – flipping from a state of hypo-arousal to hyper-arousal quickly in response to stressors. It can also take ADHDers longer to recover from stress afterwards, because

## Stressors that Render Us Vulnerable to Physical and Mental Health Challenges

| PHYSICAL STRESSORS | MENTAL STRESSORS | PSYCHOLOGICAL STRESSORS |
|---|---|---|
| Lack of sleep and rest | Time-pressured tasks | Relationship conflict |
| Noise | High standards for achievement | Loneliness |
| Excessive heat or cold | Unexpected money problems | Traumatic events |
| Overcrowding | Losing a job | Friendship challenges |
| | | Meeting expectations |

their nervous system is out of balance, which is linked to the vagus nerve. This nerve helps control automatic body functions such as breathing, heart rate and blood pressure. When the vagus nerve is working well, it's called a high vagal tone, but most ADHDers tend to have lower vagal tone, measured by heart rate variability, which reflects lower parasympathetic nervous system activity. This makes them more sensitive to tiredness and burnout. (For more on this, see Step 5, page 150.)

Additionally, many of us also have had early adverse childhood experiences (ACEs), which leave lingering traumatic imprints on our nervous system, epigenetically marking the expression of genes that are involved in various biological pathways in response to stress (see Step 4). The life we go on to have, the habits in our day to day, can be a reflection of our pre-conditioned mental states.

The good news is that there are practical things we can do right now to bring our lives back into balance, beginning with reviewing our medication, lifestyle and diet.

**Reflection**

How do you handle stress? If you were completely honest with yourself, would you say that your coping mechanisms are healthy or unhealthy? Could you replace any unhealthy habits with healthier alternatives, perhaps by spending your time and money in different ways?

## REVIEWING YOUR MEDICATION

When someone gets diagnosed with ADHD, the first line of treatment is usually medication to boost their neurotransmitter levels. However, there are a few considerations that we need to keep in mind when reviewing our medication and whether it's working for us.

- Our actual neurotype (for example, are we ADHDers or AuDHDers?), which could mean that we may not have persistently reduced levels of dopamine and norepinephrine, but rather, difficulty in regulating the right levels of these molecules.
- The prolonged sympathetic activation of our nervous system and increased stress response.
- For biological females, there will be times in our lives where fluctuations in oestrogen and progesterone can occur, which affect dopamine levels during different parts of the menstrual cycle, and during the three biggest and natural hormonal transitions in our lives – puberty, pregnancy and perimenopause (see Step 4, page 122).
- Other medications, treatments or supplements may affect our dopamine and norepinephrine levels too, such as hormone replacement therapy and vitamin B6.
- History of trauma, which can render the ADHDer more vulnerable to medication side effects.

- Some of the medications prescribed for ADHD are also used to treat binge-eating disorders, causing a tendency to forget to eat and drink.
- Our bodies can eventually develop a tolerance towards the medication, and it may become ineffective.

## Stimulants and Non-stimulants

ADHD medication options can be either stimulants or non-stimulants.

**Stimulants** are the first line of treatment for ADHD. The two main classes are methylphenidate and dextro-amphetamine, which have been used since the 1930s and come in various forms (for example, methylphenidate comes in chewable tablets, a liquid and skin patches) and acting duration (short- or long-acting). These medications increase the amount of norepinephrine and dopamine in the brain by stimulating certain cells to make more of it.

**Non-stimulants** are generally prescribed to those who don't get on with stimulants. Three non-stimulants are approved to treat ADHD: atomoxetine, guanfacine and clonidine. Atomoxetine, for example, raises frontal dopamine levels by inhibiting the protein noradrenaline transporter (NET). Clonidine and guanfacine stimulate postsynaptic and adrenergic receptors.

However, prescribing medication isn't a one and done job; they should be regularly reviewed to ensure our long-term health. Research has shown that within a year of taking the stimulant methylphenidate, for example, the brain can adjust to the increased dopamine levels by increasing the density of dopamine reuptake transporters by 24 per cent, which can cause us to suffer a more severe withdrawal effect if and when we don't want to take our medication.[7]

When the function of the dopaminergic system is changed, it doesn't end there. It can also elicit changes in the activities of downstream systems that regulate our sleep, eating habits, ability to switch gears, regulate other hormones and much more. I'm not saying all this to put you off medication. It's just that I found out the hard way that stimulants can cause adverse effects on us – and in my case, adrenal fatigue – if we don't have the knowledge and skills to manage them.

While for many ADHDers, medication can be life-changing and improve cognitive and emotional capacities, for others it may be helpful for only *a bit*, before they experience side effects. We are looking at the effects of changing the body's biochemistry, which kickstarts a cascade of activities that can lead to altered eating and sleeping patterns, as well as influencing levels of hormones that regulate various processes such as appetite suppression, stress and immune regulation, energy production, libido, the sleep–wake cycle and also thyroid function. These effects may occur in a bidirectional manner, where changes in one area influence others.

After four years of taking stimulants, I am close to learning how to optimize my medication in relation to the biology I was bestowed with, through making changes to my lifestyle and dosages across the month. However, it's important to note that everyone's body responds differently, and what works for one person may not work for another. I highly recommend reviewing your own medication and any changes with a healthcare professional to ensure you're making informed decisions based on your unique needs.

Managing your ADHD medication requires you to be mindful of what it's doing to you, the physical changes that take place in your body that can affect its effectiveness, and what daily habits and lifestyle choices are conducive to your wellbeing.

The reality is, as neurodivergents, we can be better at seeing other people's challenges than our own. When it comes to our overall physical and mental health, challenges in recognizing our own internal state, self-perception and monitoring, alexithymia (not having the words to describe our feelings and thoughts) or dyslexithymia (having the wrong words to describe them) – and then decision paralysis preventing us from doing something about it – can often lead us to repeating our behaviours.

It's helpful to work with a coach, mentor, mental health professional or community to devise holistic management strategies to ensure we can thrive with our neurodivergence.

## Risks and Benefits of ADHD Medication

| RISKS | BENEFITS |
|---|---|
| Side effects can include: headaches, nausea, dizziness, insomnia, dry mouth, higher blood pressure, appetite loss, stomach upset, anger, increased heart rate and blood pressure. | Increased quality of life, generally better mood when medication is managed and we're looking after what we eat, drink, stress levels and lifestyle. |
| Some ADHD medication can increase sensory sensitivity, making our already sensitized senses hyper-sensitive. | Better focus, ability to deal with demands and enables us to tap into our rational brain more effectively. |
| For those with pre-existing conditions such as psychosis, bipolar disorder, aggression or seizures, ADHD medications can give rise to unpredictable symptoms and may cause increased anger, suicidality, anxiety or depression. | Increased concentration on the road, which reduces motor accidents and road rage. |
| Withdrawal from ADHD medication (when taking a medication holiday) can cause depressive-like states. It's important to approach this process with professional or medical support to ensure it's done safely and effectively. | Lower likelihood of self-medicating and chasing dopamine hits with, for example, sugar, caffeine, food or casual sex when we're able to get the most out of medication. |

| RISKS | BENEFITS |
|---|---|
| Serotonin syndrome may occur when you have too much serotonin in your body, caused by taking drugs or medications that affect serotonin levels. With common symptoms including shivering and tremors, and severe symptoms including unconsciousness, this can be potentially dangerous and urgent medical care is recommended. | Women going through hormonal transitions such as perimenopause reported ADHD medication helped their symptoms. However, a holistic approach that includes hormonal therapies and lifestyle strategies should be included in treatment strategies. |
| When taken alongside other natural compounds or supplements that act as stimulants (such as ginseng, ginkgo biloba, guarana, green tea and coffee), medication can increase the levels of neurotransmitters and overstimulate the nervous system, causing anxiety, restlessness, increased heart rate, insomnia and elevated blood pressure. | Better skills to manage ADHD. For example, in therapy, having enhanced self-belief and reduced impulsivity will enable us to make better life choices. |
| When medication tapers off and results in our blood sugar levels dipping, it can cause side effects such as irritability, weepiness and anger. | Increased ability for longer-term goal-directed actions. |

## LIFESTYLE CHANGES

As we've seen, our neurodivergence can predispose us to increased sensitivity to developing many mental and physical health conditions. However, many of these conditions can be prevented if we take the first step to give our bodies what they need to scaffold our health.

The trouble with making changes to our lifestyle is that a lot of our challenges around sleep, diet, work and relationships are based on habits formed since we were young, mindsets about what fuels our self-worth, and also our traumatic beliefs.

Fundamentally, our physical needs as humans largely centre around optimizing the following:

- Nutrition
- Hydration
- Sleep
- Movement
- Oxygen intake
- Light
- Temperature
- Elimination of waste and toxins
- Balance in our health

Our neurodivergent physical needs, in the case of ADHD and autism, can also include additional needs such as:

**Homeostasis:** restoring homeostasis in a body that is prone to being in either end of an extreme state by removing unhealthy self-medicating habits first and foremost.
**Nutrition and supplementation:** replenishing our bodies with the neurotransmitters, essential nutrients, and co-factors for enzymes that are needed in many biological processes via healthier means.
**Detoxification:** reducing inflammation and toxin load.

**Hormonal changes:** being aware of our hormonal fluctuations (especially in women).
**Stress management:** having a healthier relationship with stress by managing the balance between stimulation and self-care.

When you restore optimal biological functions, you'll be surprised at how this can positively impact your executive functioning, resilience to stress, and also emotional regulation. Let's take a closer look at one of these now, which helped me recover from my present crisis: diet.

## Nutrition

Diet trumps genetics. Even if we've been born with genes that harbour mutations which lead to our genes working at altered efficiencies, we can still get a lot from our diet and supplements to help restore efficiency in these biological functions.

Here are some strategies around nutrition that the ADHD community have found helpful for their wellbeing.

1. Remember to eat at regular times and maintain blood sugar levels. Setting regular timers on your phone around meal times can help with this.
2. Choose an adequate diet of plant-based proteins containing nuts and seeds and healthy fats such as olive oil and oily fish.
3. Replenish micronutrients and amino acids that may be present at lower levels, for example vitamin B6, B12, methylated version of B9 (folate), magnesium, vitamin D, iron, l-theanine, l-tyrosine and tryptophan.
4. Prepare your gut with prebiotics and take daily probiotics to increase the diversity of healthy gut bacteria.
5. Reduce intake of or cut out inflammatory foods such as red meats, processed meats, bread and pasta made with white flour and deep-fried foods. Consume more anti-inflammatory foods like avocado, flax seeds, garlic, ginger, sweet potato, broccoli,

cabbage, blueberries, green leafy vegetables and tomatoes to reduce inflammation.
6. Maintain your blood sugar levels and energy by eating small, frequent meals, and choosing healthy snacks.
7. Cut out processed foods and eat foods that are rich in antioxidants and fibre to help your body detoxify toxins and metabolites.
8. Try plant-based oestrogens and adaptogens (herbs, roots and mushrooms that help our bodies manage stress and restore balance), for example ashwagandha, panax ginseng, lion's mane, cordyceps, turmeric and black pepper. Note that they all serve different purposes, stimulating and relaxing, so take them at different times of day to facilitate waking and sleeping times.

Remember, we are all different, so what works for one person may not work for another. For example, some neurodivergents are sensitive to dietary proteins such as gluten and lactose, or may have detoxification and inflammatory deficiencies, so it's a good idea to be mindful of what works for your personal needs. And while supplements like tyrosine may work for someone with reduced levels of dopamine, for those with fluctuating levels of it due to hormonal changes or a stressful lifestyle, for example, should consider these circumstances in their daily supplementation and nutritional needs.

### Be Proactive About Your Diet

To meet your nutritional needs, you could start now by taking action on the following:

**Genes:** Run a genetic test to find out what gene mutations you have which contribute to your behaviours, reaction to foods, drinks, medications and other substances.
**Nutritional and supplement needs:** Take your data to a clinical nutritionist or naturopath who specializes in supporting

> neurodivergents to figure out a dietary and supplementation plan to support nutritional and metabolic imbalances.
> **Gut health:** Test your gut microbiome for gut dysbiosis or mould toxicity and find out how to detoxify and replenish your gut with the good bacteria you need.
> **Bringing it all together:** Consult a health expert who is well-versed in neurodiversity to devise holistic strategies for your daily routine.
>
> When we include an adequate diet that provides the micronutrients and co-factors for enzymes that restore our biological functions to adequate proficiencies, we are taking the necessary first steps to give our body what it needs to make the most of our lives.

## NEURODIVERGENT LIFESTYLE INSIGHTS

One of our paradoxical strengths as neurodivergents is that we are able to feel more. However, in reality, when we've self-medicated with substances that affect the balance of dopamine levels or lived with a dysfunctional mindset that allowed us to repeat unhealthy coping strategies, it can be really hard to understand our authentic physical needs.

The following are lifestyle strategies informed by the collective neurodiverse community to support:

- **Self-awareness:** journaling, gratitude lists, doubling down on self-care, self-forgiveness, psychoeducation
- **Executive functioning:** body doubling (having someone present while you complete a task to aid motivation and focus), coaching, enforced breaks, flexibility, working from home, virtual assistants, pomodoro timer (breaking work into intervals with breaks in between), self-employment

- **Sleep:** consistent sleep–wake time, finding out optimal hours of sleep you need to feel good, sticking to a good sleep hygiene, afternoon naps
- **Blood sugar imbalance:** healthy protein-rich breakfasts, eating regularly, short periods between meals, meal prepping, bringing a variety of food to work, intuitive eating
- **Movement:** running, parallel play, weight training, walking, karate, marathon training, hiking
- **Regulating the nervous system:** yoga, breathwork, mindfulness, spirituality, cold water, fresh air, art, music, coffee, good tea, reading, painting and colouring by numbers, emotional freedom techniques (EFT), adaptogens
- **Light:** vitamin D, light therapy
- **Social connection:** Positive people to encourage us, social life, compassion-based therapy, community, understanding from people, counselling, remove toxic relationships

Our daily habits make us, but what works for one person may not work for another. Make sure you build the positive habits into your day to foster your health and wellbeing.

## Do Your Own Health Review

Health is not found in the extremes, so the first step in recovery is self-awareness, to be aware of what habits and mindsets no longer serve us, and replace them with a healthier alternative.

With the amount of research out there on ADHD and autism, even if it is at times gloriously terrifying, it is worth paying attention to the following factors that can tip the balance in the physiological systems in the body.

1. **Insufficient sleep:** how many hours and when do you need to sleep to feel good?

2. **Blood sugar imbalance:** how can you maintain your blood sugar level so it doesn't swing between highs and lows throughout the day?
3. **Difficult relationship with stress:** are you poor at handling stress, or swim through a stressful life unperturbed?
4. **Sedentary lifestyle:** what kind of exercises work better for you – intense exercises or a lighter version?
5. **Substance misuse:** has self-medicating with alcohol, drugs, sex, sugar, carbohydrates and other means left you feeling addicted and out of control? (See also Step 4, page 134.)
6. **Accumulation of inflammation and oxidative stress:** how is your lifestyle increasing inflammation and how can you devise strategies to reduce it?
7. **Hormonal transitions and insulin resistance:** are you at a life stage where hormonal changes can cause insulin resistance, which might exacerbate your ADHD traits by affecting your energy levels, mood and brain function?

Take a moment now to reflect on these and whether you need to address any of these areas of your life.

## LIFE STRESSORS DURING TRANSITIONS

Many of our challenges become apparent during periods of transition in our lives.

As someone who grew up in Asia and moved around the world to a country where the changes were more than cultural, I found my physical needs were affected when there were changes to:

- diet
- temperature
- availability of sunlight
- routine and lifestyle

Without knowing it, because I was heading into this life transition ill-prepared, my body and brain didn't have a chance to adapt and cope with the changes I was going through. I was in a state of prolonged stress, something I certainly felt in my body, but I wasn't aware enough of what was happening to seek help at the time.

It wasn't until I became a second-time mum that I saw the impact of my over-activated stress response on my three-month-old baby, who I was breastfeeding at the time. His dad was away for ten days, so I was effectively in sole charge of both my kids. Every one of those ten days, my baby was doing explosive green poos. If you've ever been a parent, you're told to look at your children's poo to see what's happening in their young system. As soon as my partner returned, the loose green poos stopped. The cocktail of chemicals stirred up by my stress response, which I felt in my anxiety and overwhelm, was transferred through my breastmilk into my baby boy's little gut, causing a stress response within him too.

## How to Navigate Change

How do we navigate change? You can start with these prompts:

1. Find out what is involved in the change so you can prepare for it, for example, ask for additional support to meet new demands.
2. Be aware of when the change is happening and describe it to enable yourself to process the transition.
3. Create a schedule of routine for when the transition occurs.
4. Understand your needs during the transition, for example, adequate nutrition and sleep, stress release, nutritional supplementations, community support.
5. Be aware of anxiety and stress, for example, journal both the positive things you look forward to and worries you have about the change.

## Know Your Limits

At the end of the day, it really comes down to knowing the limits of your energy levels. It's so important to create a buffer between taking on a project and passing the point of no return – burnout. For many neurodivergents, burnout can look like depression, and in fact the ICD-11 (International Classification of Diseases) has gone as far as classifying burnout under a clinical diagnosis of depression. The state of burnout for neurodivergents can create a neurotoxic effect where its impact can be felt in the entire body.

It's important to understand that even if we do inherit gene variants that can predispose us to ADHD, autism, mental and physical health conditions, this doesn't mean that any of these are definitely going to manifest in disease. Differences in these genes mean that the proteins work with altered efficiency – perhaps they are underactive, overactive, or lacking the mechanisms required to regulate their levels.

However, we need not despair. Although we can't change the genes we've inherited, we can change how they are expressed. Genes may deal us our cards in the game of life, but it's how we play the hand that we're dealt that counts.

As neurodivergents, our way of being can be likened to being handed the controller to the game of our life. The instruction manual is imprinted in your genes, and while you couldn't control your early nurture or change the past, it is up to you to press the buttons and steer the ship from here on. If you know that you have increased sensitivities to the factors that I mention in this chapter, how do you want to proceed in this game now?

As we will see in Step 4, while we can't change which genes we've inherited, we can influence the ways in which they are expressed. Genes are mutable by virtue of their nature. And we can also begin to understand how our past experiences and circumstances have shaped the ways in which they play out in our lives.

# Step 4:
# Trace Your Beginnings

You made it Earth side. This is where everything that nature intended will rear its head in the life you lead from here. Yes, your genes are loaded in your system, raring to go since your entry into the world, but what determines whether these genes are actually expressed, and if they are, in what way?

In this fourth Step, we are going to explore the next level of the ADHD iceberg, which is about the ways in which our family and culture can influence how our neurodiverse traits manifest themselves. Along the way, we will also be looking at other important factors, such as race and gender – including how our hormones can interact with our ADHD if we are biologically female.

### LOOKING UNDER THE MICROSCOPE

When I studied molecular biology, genetics, microbes, immune system and cancer, I was fascinated by the behaviour of cells and how a single unit like a cell can house multiple factories and warehouses that perform so many different functions – to power up, self-duplicate and transport the right molecules to kickstart the many programmes that keep us alive. This process, when it works, paints a picture of health and vitality. But it is not always seamless, as it can change according to the cues our cells receive from their internal and external environments.

My introduction to cell-to-cell communication took place when I looked at how bacterial cells talk to one another through sensing chemical signals released by neighbouring cells. To perform a colony-wide function, they need to sense a critical mass or density, known as a 'quorum', before they can switch on or off genes that enable them to do things like become infectious, form biofilms or create bioluminescence.

While working in cancer research, I was struck by what happened when we put healthy cells next to the damaged ones. When I grew healthy human cells on top of cells that were damaged by gamma radiation in the lab, I observed that the healthy human cells began showing DNA damage, indicated by a significant increase in a protein produced in response to this damage. This led me to postulate that the damaged cells communicated with the healthy cells via chemicals released into the in-between spaces, altering the gene expression in the healthy cells.

In other words, these simple experiments showed me that our cells are responsive to environmental cues, subsequently altering their expression of genes, proteins and downstream biological processes. In our human bodies, the picture is more complex; the behavioural outcome of cells (and therefore the way we develop and function) is subject to many factors, including:

- Internal environmental cues. For example gender, hormones and metabolism.
- External environmental cues. For example diet, temperature, oxygen levels, humidity, light, presence of mutagens or stressors, drugs, toxins and chemicals.
- The ways different cells communicate and the substrates involved. For example brain cells can communicate through chemical and electrical signals, while gut cells can communicate through mechanical signals (such as the stretching of the stomach to signal feeling full).

Seeing how malleable our cells are, it makes sense that we are wired to adapt to our environment, for better or for worse. An understanding of this can help set the stage for discussing the roles that nature and nurture play in shaping our neurodiverse experiences and innate differences.

## HOW DO OUR GENES PLAY OUT?

What causes the mutations in genes that give rise to such diverse sets of functions in large groups of people? To understand the genetics of ADHD and other forms of neurodivergence that predispose us to certain traits, we need to understand how gene evolution works.

Genes that appeared fewer than 10–30 million years ago are considered good models when studying the early evolution of genes, to understand what shaped their origins and how their structures and functions developed. This period goes all the way back to the Cenozoic era, when early humans first started walking on two legs, signifying the dawn of human evolution, when large scale adaptations to life in nature began.[1]

In the context of evolution, many genes are conserved in the genetic lineage due to the process of natural selection, as the environment we live in calls for the continuous expression of those traits that enable us to survive there. Given that is so, we might wonder whether there is any genetic advantage to inheriting the traits associated with ADHD.

In his book *ADHD: A Hunter in a Farmer's World*,[2] Thom Hartmann writes that ADHD is far too ubiquitous for it to be a 'mistake'. Hartmann sees ADHD as a natural way of being that descended from a long line of hunters who adapted to behave in ways that suited the times when humans had to forage for wild produce and hunt for food. In fact, a study published in *Nature* magazine in 2020 looked into the ancestral origins of ADHD and found gene variants linked to ancestral traits of ADHD.[3] The study supported the role of natural selection pressures on the early-onset functions implicated in ADHD. A more recent study by Dr David Barack's team at the University of Pennsylvania also seems to confirm Hartmann's theory by suggesting that ADHD traits such as distractibility and impulsivity may have been an evolutionary advantage for our ancestors, as these may have improved their tactics when exploring and foraging for food.[4]

I can't imagine how stressful it must have been for our distant ancestors to remain constantly alert so they could run for safety in a moment's notice, or take it in turns to stand guard at night when there were likely to be dangers everywhere. However, I can imagine that our genes would need to evolve to create neural structures that enable us to feel more, sense danger, think less, and mobilize quicker – reactions that are synonymous with the fight-or-flight response.

Natural selection meant that possessing the traits that worked in the hunter-gatherer days could still work in later eras to an extent, depending on individual contexts. The traits such as sensation- and novelty-seeking needed to be adapted to life in a more ordered society. If this was channelled towards invention and exploration that benefit humanity, it would be deemed as useful, but less so if these traits were channelled towards hedonistic pursuits, which could potentially end in disaster. As the centuries rolled on and society increasingly became more organized, perhaps some ADHDers were indeed able to camouflage themselves as inventors and scientists, while others undoubtedly fell through the rungs of society. For example, although ADHD made it hard for Einstein to buckle down and sit tight in a classroom at university when he had a roving mind that valued autonomy and creativity, neurodivergence served him well when he came up with the Theory of Relativity during a year out satisfying his itch to travel.

Ultimately, whether a trait is retained depends on whether the society we live in enables it to be passed along to the next generation; it may not matter whether it is more beneficial or harmful, it just is. Researchers have found that the gene variants that on the whole increase one's ADHD susceptibility have steadily decreased since Palaeolithic times, supporting the hypothesis that modern society is applying negative selective pressure against ADHD-risk variants.[5] The evolving world has enabled large-scale gene adaptations which appear to be gradually phasing out those variants that are deemed destructive and retaining those that are socially beneficial.

However, we also need to be aware that historical events such as war, forced migration, famine, slavery, ethnic cleansing, racism, rise of capitalism, poverty, advent of innovation, worldwide pandemics and the age of AI have all brought us here. Some of these events were catastrophic and traumatic and have left their imprint on future generations. Although these sorts of experiences won't necessarily have mutated your great-grandparents' or parents' genes, they may still work through a number of ways – such as inducing the stress response, eliciting downstream biological processes, and changing the way the gene is read via a mechanism known as epigenetics. The latter changes gene expression and functions over a few generations. This is why it's likely that before you were even born, generational trauma may have become etched into your cellular programme. But it isn't all bad news: epigenetics takes into account the effects of our environment on our genes. This means that as well as nature, nurture and lifestyle have a very important role to play in how our ADHD expresses itself in our lives. While we can't change our past or our upbringing, we can change our thinking and our attitudes in ways that will improve our wellbeing.

Of course, that means that we too have an active part to play. We can sometimes become so focused on the label and its related traits that it distracts us from recognizing the everyday habits and actions that may be contributing to our ill health. And that's why we need to become aware of our own mindset.

## UNDERSTAND YOUR MINDSET

As somebody with ADHD, I'm no stranger to the general perception that women like me can look like inattentive day dreamers. We are the graceful swans who are paddling vigorously below the water. Under the veneer of perfectionism that we carefully construct, we are desperate for help. If only we knew how to ask for it.

As I went through the biggest transition in my life, a divorce while co-parenting two kids, my environment changed completely. I'd yet to find ways to cope while the demands piled up around me. Emails and messages that spilled in became a source of anxiety; it was impossible to deal with a business that was growing amid the storm I was in. I became sleep deprived from focusing on everyone and everything else but me.

I was so hung up on the ideas around the biological systems that were going wrong inside me that I forgot the biggest culprit – my mindset.

Three years into taking my ADHD medication, and with no medication review until two and a half years into it, I lost 8kg in weight. At 46kg, I was lighter than my teenage self. My life was chaotic, I was overworked, and I lost my appetite while I was on the ADHD medication and mostly skipped lunch. I began to experience mid-afternoon blood sugar crashes, and there came a point when my medication was only working for two or three hours a day.

The tide turned when my friend Dr Bernadette Dancy got in touch and threw me a lifeline in the form of health coaching. I know it sounds ridiculous that even with her amazing offer for support, the first thing that came into my mind was, 'Where will I find the time for this?' My health was on the line, help was at hand, and yet I initially rejected it. Bernie said to me, 'While you are doing all these talks supporting other neurodivergents, who's looking after Sam?'

I'm not sharing this story because I want sympathy – quite the opposite. You can know all the right things to do, yet you still don't do them. Today, I want to show up better and walk the talk, so now I follow my own advice on neurodiversity and wellbeing. And hopefully my experience will help you see that you may have some pre-conditioned beliefs that are harming you more than helping you.

## THE IMPORTANCE OF REVISITING YOUR BELIEFS

It wasn't until I read the amazing *ADDitude* magazine article 'Women with ADHD: No More Suffering in Silence' written by Ellen Littman that I felt really seen.[6] The things I overlooked were largely fed by the beliefs that I'm not entitled to a support system, but that I *am* the support system. Being the person who initiated my divorce, I felt responsible for my children's and ex-husband's challenges. I took it all upon myself to hold the fort and be the steadying factor for everyone. But I really wasn't a steady fort, more like a sinking fort. I was constantly overwhelmed and frantic trying to go from one place to another and barely meeting the demands that ruled my life.

But slowly, things got better. My amazing colleague and friend Catherine and I finally found a way to help reduce the overwhelm I was experiencing from my business. She even helped me create a co-parenting schedule and told me that it's okay to lock in the weekends to spend time with my children so the schedule would be fairer and there'd also be time for respite. I don't know why, but I always look to other people like Catherine to give me the permission to do something that appears 'selfish', even when it's nothing more than an act of self-preservation.

When Bernie and I eventually sat down and chatted for the first time, I still had persistent brain fog and anxiety. My breathing issues were better, but it was as though my heart had retained a memory of its struggles, and my breathing was still quite shallow. I had trouble sleeping, often tossing and turning through the night.

But the biggest revelation was that a lot of my health issues originated from ignoring a very simple basic life habit – one you need to do every day, if you want to stay alive. I needed to start eating nutritious meals each day to give my brain and body the fuel they needed, and I needed to drink pure $H_2O$. By neglecting to both eat and drink, I was going into my days in an energy-deficit mode, essentially introducing prolonged famine in my body.

This is why I say that you can know all the right things to do, yet you don't do them.

## Neurodivergent Challenges

As a neurodivergent, you may have challenges around:

- Beliefs and conditioning that make you pour your energy outward instead of inward.
- Other co-occurring forms of neurodivergence or physical or mental health conditions, which complicate your perception of what's truly happening.
- The medication working differently for you, so you become overfocused and have trouble switching gears, hence forgetting about everything else.
- Unhealthy coping strategies that are distorting your work–life balance, eventually harming your health.
- Being unaware of what's happening in your body until it's too late and you begin showing the symptoms.
- Being unable to whittle your situation down to one thing to act on.
- Feeling overloaded by too much information and not knowing what specifically helps you.

Besides nature, nurture has a big role in shaping the unique you. If we were to put a neurodivergent brain in a vacuum, deprived of feedback from its internal and external environment, neurodivergence is likely to be shaped by what is programmed to happen. But all that changes when we expose the brain to a life of significant stimulation. Neuroplasticity is a concept where new synapses are fired as a result of our interaction with the environment that we live in, forming new neural pathways.

Before we are even born, our early experiences in the womb, including exposure to any allergens, stressors, toxins or even infections, can influence whether, when and how our genes release the instructions that build our future capacity for health, skills and resilience. Our experiences in utero also have the ability to mark our genes chemically, generating epigenetic signatures that activate or dampen our genetic potential.

Moreover, while some neurodivergent traits and even generational trauma are loaded into our cellular programme, they may only be 'notes' we've inherited, not necessarily fixed characteristics, and may be rewritten by our own life experiences and actions. Let's start by considering how you were responded to from birth.

## ADHD AND EARLY CHILDHOOD EXPERIENCES

In his best-selling book *They F\*\*\* You Up*,[7] clinical psychologist Oliver James summarized how the ways we are cared for in the first six years of life fundamentally affect who we are and how we behave. When we are born, we rely on our parents and caregivers to provide us with what we need and to regulate our emotions. We automatically seek attachment. This will go really well if we have well-adjusted parents who can be there for us, or at least able to outsource the parenting to more reliable caregivers if not. But sadly, that's not always the case.

In a poll done within the ADHD Girls community in 2021, all but one person out of over 100 respondents said that they encountered adverse childhood experiences (ACEs). I later asked the only person who said they didn't encounter childhood trauma about her experiences when growing up, and she told me, 'There wasn't any obvious trauma. Yes, there was invalidation, and I was left to cry on my own when I felt dysregulated, but I won't call that trauma.' But emotional neglect like this is trauma, where there wasn't anyone to validate and help this respondent to make sense of her emotions. If we are left to navigate these huge emotions by ourselves, we may never really learn how to do this successfully by ourselves.

Many ADHDers had experienced ACEs, social deprivation and intergenerational trauma. Chaos often surrounds a household in these scenarios. Our parents might have shown unhealthy emotional and behavioural patterns or perhaps didn't show up at all for us, causing potential attachment ruptures early in our lives. Is it any wonder that fewer than ten per cent of kids with ADHD have secure attachment styles?[8] Many go on to develop an anxious-avoidant attachment style, which can challenge their ability to regulate their emotions in their relationships with others (see Step 6 for more on attachment styles).[9] Studies have also shown that exposure to four or more ACEs is associated with lower health outcomes and higher incidence of ADHD and mental health challenges.[10]

But it's not all doom and gloom. Perhaps, just perhaps, God is fair. Some of us may have been lucky to have had experiences that increase our resilience in the face of life's challenges. A study found promising results when it looked into individual, family and community resilience as factors that balance out the effect of ACEs.[11] It was discovered that among children with four or more ACEs, individual resilience decreased their chances of developing mental health challenges; community resilience through stress management and mindfulness practices decreased depression (with individual resilience resulting in the strongest protective effect); and family resilience, where a parent engaged with their child and supported them, significantly diminished the effect of ACEs on mental, emotional and behavioural conditions.[12]

As I contemplated this, it dawned on me that the reasons I was able to get back up each time I was knocked down were due to many of the positive experiences I'd encountered in my life. Despite having had more than four ACEs, I was lucky to have developed the self-belief in my abilities through being acknowledged and nurtured for my skills and interests in athletics, sports and biology; self-awareness by journaling throughout my teen years; healthy eating; and having good teachers and friends who were good influences on me.

If you've managed to fly under the radar for most of your life, there's a really good chance you've internalized a lot of your challenges, or that, like me, you've had a good support system around you. You may have always known you were different, but because you've been so busy adapting to look like everyone else, perhaps you couldn't tell what was an innate part of your nature, and what had been shaped by the life you've led and society around you.

> ### Resilience in ADHD Children
>
> Research shows that the following can be protective factors that help promote resilience in children with ADHD.[13] These are the 'antidotes' for those who have experienced ACEs.
>
> **Your family gets along:** knowing you can talk to your family about your feelings and there's someone in your home who keeps you safe.
>
> **Positive parenting skills:** healthy emotional understanding and practical guidance.
>
> **Positive social contact:** having friends who care about you, being an active participant in your school group, having a role in community traditions, having two non-parental adults who take a genuine interest in you.
>
> **Self-concept of strengths:** understanding ADHD-associated strengths, believing you are competent, possess strong cognitive abilities and effectively utilize them, good self-esteem, character strengths of being optimistic, hopeful, grateful and zestful, and have self-regulation skills.
>
> **Interpersonal skills:** being able to control emotions and behaviours in social situations.

## HOW CULTURE INTERACTS WITH ADHD

When I look at the differences in the way our neurodivergence manifest across different cultures, communities and life circumstances, one thing becomes glaringly obvious: our place in society largely determines our chances. Some of our stories are truly written in the stars: the places we began and where we are now, the chances we are given, the privilege and bias/oppression we experience based on how we are viewed by others all shape our neurodiverse experience.

As neurodivergents, we don't begin life on a level playing field and we then go on to be conditioned by both the parenting we receive and by the distinct cultural rules of the society we belong to. Socially, there are notable parallels between the experiences of neurodivergent individuals and those who identify with intersectionality. 'Intersectionality' is a term coined by law professor Kimberlé Crenshaw in 1989 that refers to the complex and cumulative way that the effects of different forms of discrimination (such as racism, sexism and classism) can overlap, interact and affect people. Similarly, individuals who have neurological differences such as ADHD, ASD, dyslexia and co-occurring conditions often face challenges stemming from societal discrimination, stigma and misunderstanding. Just as intersectionality recognizes the unique experience that comes from dealing with multiple forms of discrimination, being neurodivergent typically involves confronting various forms of bias and exclusion.

In both cases, the individuals affected must navigate systems that, due to a lack of awareness, understanding or accommodation, often marginalize and disadvantage them. Both neurodivergents and those at the intersection of various identities (such as gender, disability, race, ethnicity, class and gender identity) have unique experiences that cannot be fully understood if considering their identities in isolation. Therefore, it's essential to take an inclusive and intersectional approach when thinking about neurodiversity – as often individuals will inhabit multiple identities at once.

If I think about the lives of intersectional neurodivergents as a process, when we are born, our parents raise us via their own internalized cultural norms and beliefs, which changes our biology right away. Our early environment embeds biological 'memories' in our neurodevelopment, affects the development of our body's stress response systems, shaping our brain structures, heart, immune response, digestive and metabolic regulatory systems. It also has an impact that persists far into adulthood and leads to lifelong changes to our physical and mental health.

As intersectional neurodivergents grow up in their respective cultures, their personalities are further shaped according to the values that are upheld in their place in society. They react in the following ways.

- Follow the 'societal rules' playbook given to their unique identity.
- Have unique ways of internalizing challenges they face, based on what is expected and normalized.
- Develop coping strategies that are deemed as acceptable within their distinct cultures.
- Not see maladaptive behaviours as a problem because their culture does not define them as one.
- Not have the words or know how to ask for help.

And do you know who this affects?

Just about everyone, other than the dominant culture in society. When I say 'dominant culture', I'm referring to a group of people with a specific way of being that society is made for, where the systems support their attainment or health and wealth, and fulfilment of potential. When society is made for a dominant way of being, everyone else who doesn't fit into that specific identity is at risk of being marginalized and therefore needs to adapt or risk being ostracized.

When we zoom down to the cellular level, the trauma internalized by an underrepresented group who've had a history of intergenerational oppression cannot be separated from that experienced by being a neurodivergent alone. The overlapping social identities compound the trauma, leading to yet more challenges in our identification of a problem, seeking community, and our recovery.

Resmaa Menakem, an author and psychotherapist who specializes in the effects of trauma on the human body, says, 'Trauma decontextualized in a people over time can look like culture'.[14] If I were to add to her words, I would say we interact with the people and events that come into our lives, adapting to experiences that induce neuroplasticity, creating behaviours and motivations that look outwardly like personality. When we have children, we project this personality onto our family members, which can then become family traits that are embedded in our children as they internalize the trauma. Over time, this way of being becomes shared, especially if many in the society begin to act in the same ways, which are then ultimately accepted as a cultural norm.

Besides my own experiences as a Southeast Asian woman with ADHD who lives in the UK, I've embraced learning about our collective hidden experiences through launching my podcast campaign Utopia, in which I interview neurodivergents across different communities and life circumstances from different gender, race, religion, disability, social class and migrant status backgrounds. What I unearthed was awe-inspiring, through courageous conversations with intersectional neurodivergents who had had to adapt so they could get ahead, to swim so they need not sink, to stay safe or alive. As so much of my work is with women with ADHD, I'd like us to take a look next at the role that gender plays in the ways that our ADHD manifests itself.

## GENDER AND ADHD

I'm often asked about the differences in gender presentations of ADHD. While it's generally believed that men with ADHD tend to present with externalizing behaviours such as hyperactive-impulsive, substance misuse, conflict avoidance to anger outbursts, and having low frustration tolerance, women with ADHD are largely seen as inattentive, day dreamers, anxious and depressed people-pleasers.

This is what drove me to create my first iceberg picture for women with ADHD, shown in Step 1, to go beneath the surface and see what is at play. For example, if an undiagnosed neurodivergent woman presents as chaotic and emotionally dysregulated in the doctor's office because she's going through a relationship break-up while in perimenopause, on the surface this may look like anxiety or depression. If she is presumed to have a history of trauma, a reliance on drinking and drugs, then an additional assessment such as mood disorder, post-traumatic stress disorder (PTSD) or borderline personality disorder (BPD) may be carried out. However, her doctor might not think about neurodivergence as a possibility right away because there are so many layers to whittle through and most people don't make it past the surface of our observable behaviours. And even when ADHD or autism is considered, the challenge lies in the lack of training for medical professionals on the women-specific manifestations of neurodivergence.

By the time a neurodivergent woman gets around to seeking support, she's often already developed archetypical personality traits (see the box below). Beneath, though, we're also looking at two contributing factors to the archetypes – the effects of socialization over a lifetime, and our internal biological states.

---

### Archetypal Personality Traits of Neurodivergent Women

- Perfectionist
- High achiever
- Burned out
- People-pleaser
- Independent
- Feisty and loud
- Class clown
- Nurturing, at the expense of her own needs
- Need to control
- Demand for high standard
- Stressed
- Self-critical

---

**Reflection**

Today, part of my work involves supporting late-diagnosed neurodivergent women who come to me looking for effective strategies to manage their lives with ADHD, whether it's support relating to work, career, or building the skills to manage their medication. Ultimately, I find it's often our mindset that needs to be addressed. I tend to steer the conversation back to the underlying issues.

I'd like you to take a moment now to consider this question, too: 'If you have or are seeking an ADHD diagnosis, what are you hoping to improve in your life?'

## THE EFFECT OF FEMALE HORMONES

Compared to male biology, a woman's hormone levels tend to ebb and flow more dramatically in each month of her fertile years, when the balance between oestrogen and progesterone changes. In addition to this, major fluctuations in her hormones occur during distinct milestones in her life, such as puberty, pregnancy, after childbirth and during perimenopause. These major hormonal changes are completely natural processes, but can come with distinct challenges.

Neurodivergent women face an added layer of complexity, because we're dealing with the impact of these hormonal fluctuations on a system that already doesn't always work in sync. Then, when we experience mysterious symptoms such as cognitive challenges, mood swings and sleep disturbances, we may become even more perplexed and doubt ourselves.

Oestrogen, it turns out, is the master regulator of women's brain health. The neuroscientist Dr Lisa Mosconi studied the menopausal brain and found that there is distinct brain remodelling taking place at this crucial transition – our brains are actually changing in structure, connectivity and energy metabolism.[15] During menopause, the remodelling that takes place has a strong impact on mood, cognition, sleep and stress resilience as this transition stage is prompted by the brain. As neurodivergent and intersectional identities are known to enter menopause at a younger than average age, this means we can face these difficulties earlier than expected.[16,17]

We know that oestrogen indirectly regulates dopamine, and for many of us neurodivergent women, dopamine is like a distant, unreliable friend who displays both hot and cold personas. So, when oestrogen is high, dopamine tends to increase, and women with ADHD tend to show risk-taking and impulsive behaviours. When oestrogen is low, dopamine swiftly dips, in addition to serotonin and acetylcholine, leaving us with cognitive difficulties, mood challenges and sleep issues.[18]

Many neurodivergent women also experience a more severe form of premenstrual syndrome, known as premenstrual dysphoric disorder (PMDD). Although the exact biochemical causes of PMDD is not yet known, there have been studies showing that women with PMDD tend to experience more drastic symptoms when the balance between oestrogen and progesterone changes throughout the month. While there could be other root causes for hormonal imbalances, one of the most effective ways to recovery is to manage your stress.

From a physiological context, hormonal fluctuations may render neurodivergent women more susceptible to challenges around executive functioning, controlling emotions in daily interactions, the ability to think rationally, reason with our inner critic, sleep, and be resilient to relational stresses. This is because the hormone oestrogen impacts dopamine, acetylcholine and serotonin – the neurotransmitters that control our motivation, working memory, behavioural self-regulation, sleep, emotional regulation, time management, organization, stress management, wellbeing and happiness.

Imagine the chaos caused by not knowing this at every big hormonal transition in your life, beginning at puberty through to menopause. If you're biologically female and reading this, let that realization dawn upon you: how many situations you've unwittingly gone into ill-prepared and the cost this has had on your mental and emotional health.

The literature is now flooded with anecdotal and empirical evidence that neurodivergent women with ADHD and autism see a worsening of their traits with fluctuations in their oestrogen and progesterone levels.[19] This begins from puberty and continues to affect us through our monthly cyclical fluctuation of sex hormones, which can be divided into four phases in our cycle. I like to compare these to four different seasons of moods (the following table is intended only for guidance. There is no one way for a woman to experience her menstrual cycle):

**Spring (Day 6–11):** Early follicular phase – and a time for starting projects and working on ideas, being motivated and exercising to release energy.

**Summer (Day 12–18):** Follicular phase, ovulation and early luteal phase – and a time for focus, verbal articulation, more energy for social connections, higher intensity exercises, good sleep and diet. Drop in hormones straight after ovulation warrants more self-care.

**Autumn (19–25):** Early to late luteal phase – and a time for aligning with the truth, rest, talking about relationship needs and boundaries, detoxifying, reducing stress, lower intensity exercises, adequate diet and sleep.

**Winter (Day 26–28, 1–5):** Late luteal, menstruation phase – and a time for rest, integrating ideas, listening to your body, avoid strong exercise, detoxify and reflection.

Towards ovulation, increasing levels of oestrogen enhance our neurotransmitters such as dopamine, acetylcholine and serotonin, improving cognitive functioning and affecting risk-taking and reward-seeking behaviours. This is followed by a drop in oestrogen after ovulation and in the lead-up to menstruation, which can have a negative effect, resulting in avoidant behaviours and reduced executive functioning.[20] Oestrogen's decline can cause mental, emotional, sensory and social-communication challenges, but the role it plays on other organs such as our heart, bones, brain, liver, colon and skin can lead to longer-term physical health challenges if we aren't able to tackle the problem at its source.

On top of this, other procedures that dramatically change the hormonal levels in a neurodivergent woman's life can also increase our vulnerability to unforeseen challenges. These include but aren't limited to the procedure of egg freezing, in vitro fertilization, cancer treatment, and many other procedures. And that's before we've even taken into account the social pressures on women!

## How Do Your Hormones Interact with Your ADHD?

If you are biologically female, to get a clearer picture of how your own hormones might be affecting the way that your ADHD manifests, you can start by doing a life audit.

- Are you experiencing any major hormonal transitions, such as puberty, pregnancy, postpartum, perimenopause or menopause?
- Do you notice changes in mood, sleep, energy levels, libido and cognitive ability across the month (if you have a regular menstrual cycle)?
- Are your life demands and stressors interfering with your ability to reduce stress, thereby potentially impacting your body's ability to balance your hormones?
- Look back to the sections on diet and lifestyle at the end of Step 3: does your body have what it needs to function optimally?
- Are there times in your cycle when ADHD medication feels stronger or weaker?

This approach can be a start to you balancing your hormones.

1. Track your menstrual cycle, being aware of when to expect changes in your sex hormones and adjust your activities accordingly. For example, do social activities when you have more energy and feel verbally articulate, and ensure you get adequate rest when you are approaching menstruation.
2. Reduce stress and demands by setting boundaries and employ stress-busting strategies such as practising yoga or Pilates or going for gentle walks in nature.

3. Reduce exposure to xenoestrogens. These are environmental chemicals – found for example in plastics and personal care products that contain parabens or pesticides – that your body may think are real oestrogen, and will therefore make less of the real thing.
4. Make dietary changes to provide your body and brain with what they need to balance your hormones. Add healthy fats to your diet, eat proteins with every meal, include leafy greens and cruciferous vegetables to increase oestrogen detoxification, limit refined sugars to avoid blood sugar spikes and stay hydrated to support metabolic and hormonal function.
5. Aim for 20–45 minutes of daily exercise and movement – even short bursts count! Mix it up based on your energy and focus levels, from low impact (walking) or moderate (cycling, dance), to high intensity (HIIT) and strength training.
6. Focus on sorting out your sleep hygiene and getting the right amount of sleep you need to feel rested, regulated and re-energized.
7. Supplement your diet as appropriate.

## THE SOCIALIZATION OF GIRLS

The society we grow up in usually has preconceived ideas of what is considered appropriate for girls. And this appears to change subtly across generations and borders. As a millennial who grew up being told that she should be seen and not heard, that she can be 'too much' and that her thoughts were often 'too far out', I was often confused about the double standards that seemed to be applied to me.

Typically, as neurodivergent girls grow up to be women, we often have to deal with:

- Hiding our authentic needs to behave in the ways that are expected of a 'good girl'.
- Developing coping strategies that can border on obsession, appearing 'all or nothing', trying harder and self-chastising when we can't engage.
- Potentially self-medicating to manage societal demands for communication and cooperation, while dealing with unpredictable executive function caused by hormonal fluctuations.
- Instead of seeking support for ourselves, becoming a support for others.
- Self-censorship due to shame related to our issues with emotional regulation.[21]
- Needing to appear perfect, to avoid disappointing others and ourselves.
- Not having the words or know how to ask for help, leading to misdiagnosis of anxiety, depression, PMDD, BPD or mood disorders.
- Increasing demands as we age (juggling motherhood and career, caring responsibilities).
- A changing landscape in our brains, hormones and bodies, while questioning our ability to meet demands, instead of our biology and self-care.
- Keeping up with the façade.

When I became a mother, I felt stifled by the immediate expectations others had of me. I had to breastfeed because that was thought to be the best option for my child, so I set an alarm to wake up every two hours while I was recovering from natural childbirth. It's not that I didn't want to do any of these things, but more that I felt that everyone around me expected me to do this despite how much I was struggling. Because I was exclusively breastfeeding by the time my daughter turned one, I felt that I was all my daughter had. If I'd had more support (or permission to be more selfish) at the time and received more compassion and felt less shame around what I was going through, perhaps I wouldn't have developed debilitating postnatal anxiety and depression that made it hard for me to go back to work. Perhaps I wouldn't have viewed the situation via an 'all or nothing' lens. If I felt there were more capable hands who did the job as good as I did, I would have been less rigid, less controlling; I would have allowed some flexibility. I would have been able to reach out for help.

Just when do we hold up the flag and say enough is enough? Understanding what we need to show up as our healthier, authentic selves is the first step towards thriving. The hardest part for so many neurodivergent women, despite knowing the right thing to do at times, is the messaging we've internalized from people around us, such as our partners, colleagues and systems in society. With so many neurodivergent women being diagnosed with ADHD and autism later in life when perimenopause symptoms surface, we're only now finding out that part of the problem wasn't us.

It is largely because of these internalized beliefs that we hide our challenges, or what others call our impairments, when in fact, we've been told 'the right way' to behave from day one. These societal beliefs are so normalized that as women, we play our parts in reinforcing the stereotypical female roles that cause so many neurodivergent women to struggle needlessly and be misunderstood, misdiagnosed and mistreated.[22]

In childhood, the ratio of girls to boys diagnosed with ADHD is between 1:3 and 1:16, depending on the country. In adulthood, this ratio equalizes at 1:1. While more boys are diagnosed with hyperactivity and impulsivity, more girls reach out for emotional and mood challenges, with 14 per cent of girls with ADHD being prescribed antidepressants before being treated for ADHD, compared to only 5 per cent of boys.[23]

What does this internalized sense of never meeting the expectations of others look like? It's found in the ways we women beat ourselves up for our 'shortcomings', how we've always wanted to be autonomous, but we were told our authentic needs are not important or welcomed. Over time, it can feel like the system is trying to control us – slowly silencing our voice and making it harder to express what we truly need.

If we haven't learned to honour our needs, we believe that as long as we are able to give others what they need from us – in so far as we are useful, compliant and able to meet others' expectations – we are okay. But we are not okay. And it is high time we emerge from the layers of conditioning that make us neglect ourselves, even if this neglect has a root. And if the fact of being a woman were not enough of a complication in obtaining a diagnosis for ADHD, it's not made any easier by other factors over which we have little to no control.

## RACE, ETHNICITY AND CLASS

When you strip it all back, if society is made for a dominant culture, is it any wonder that the ones who are most vocal about their needs and are able to express them will be heeded first? While we ADHDers may all face similar innate challenges, those who were born in cultures that exert harsh punishments on misbehaviour and praise for qualities such as endurance are likely to want to hide their challenges even further.

I was someone who masked her neurodivergence because I grew up in Asia during a time in history that did not welcome individuality. There were certain qualities that were deemed to be culturally acceptable, such as being an achiever, whether in sports or academics – which I took to so naturally I remember being surprised by it.

As the oldest girl in a family of five children, I was praised for being the 'easy child'. I was told 'don't cry' every time I did. I was also commended for being able to tolerate pain and not complain, which I saw as a strength. As I grew up, I knew it was possible to hide my hyperactivity, but it turned into fatigue and anxiety. I also knew it was possible to hide my inability to understand verbal instructions and process them in real time by watching carefully what my friends were doing. I remember when I had to copy my friends' work, because I didn't understand what was being asked of us.

So, later in university, when I was called a 'genius', I didn't believe it at all. Because everything I'd achieved was based on sheer hard work to manage a brain that constantly wanted to go against the plans I made for it. And my anxiety has never left me, because I never know when my brain will decide it doesn't want to play ball.

The inability to voice my needs has followed me all the way through to . . . now. The need to comply didn't serve me when I failed to say no when I was groomed as a student, and when I got into relationships because others chose me – it didn't seem to matter if I liked them or not.

But how do you tell your doctor that these are the symptoms of your neurodivergence? The internal chastising that never leaves you? The negative thoughts that keep going round in your head on a loop? The impending sense of danger that is never too far away? The persistent sense of fear that never leaves when you're doing life alone? How do you explain the way neurodivergence shows up for you if it doesn't look anything like what's discussed in medical journals, books or social media?

Evelyn Polk Green, past president of the Attention Deficit Disorder Association (called ADDA for short), was one of my favourite interviewees in my Utopia campaign. Her warrior quality shone through from her work supporting neurodivergents from underrepresented and impoverished backgrounds. In my interview with her, she courageously remarked upon how meekly polite her black kids were compared to her friends' white boys when they went into a supermarket: 'If my kids behave that way, that'll get them dead.' It was a sentence that shook me to the core, as I had been unaware of my own privilege up until that point.

As an Asian woman, to the world I was largely seen as hardworking, polite and productive. I do as I am told, work hard and swallow my feelings. I'm not saying that this is true, it's just what I have always felt was expected of me. So, when I was asked by an Asian corporate client, 'Why isn't there a single Asian person in the neurodiversity employee resource group in our company?' I replied by saying, 'Because you don't know how neurodivergence manifests for you.'

Given the rules that we've all been playing by and the expectations that we are meant to behave in ways that are deemed appropriate by our culture, and as we are guided by different cultural values, is it any wonder our neurodivergence manifests differently? As we saw in Step 1, the diagnostic criteria for all neurodivergence and mental health conditions were based traditionally on research done on white boys. It is gender-, culture-, race- and wholly biased. And if diagnosis and support are tailored to neurodivergence characteristics displayed by a naughty white boy (in the case of ADHD), then we are missing the right strategies for supporting adults, women and those with other identities.

So how does ADHD and autism manifest clinically in a culture where people are applauded for their ability to hold back tears, eat stress for breakfast, not complain and try harder? Gabor Maté said in an interview with Steven Bartlett that in all his years of medical practice, he has found that the people who develop autoimmune and chronic diseases are the ones who hold back their feelings and are most concerned about pleasing others.[24]

We also know that when stress can't be released in healthy ways, it manifests as long-term chronic stress, or burnout. It manifests in physical symptoms such as headaches, brain fog, anxiety, panic attacks, chest pain, menstrual changes and gut, adrenal and immune system issues.[25] If neurodivergents from global majority groups aren't showing up as forgetful, disruptive or impulsive, you bet we're showing up with physical ailments and emotional dysregulation that we often find difficult to explain to anyone, let alone ourselves.

So how do people from different cultural identities cope with stress?

Naturally, we do it via ways that are deemed as acceptable by the culture we find ourselves in or that has formed us. In the same way that drinking alcohol and smoking marijuana is normalized in many Western societies, there are Eastern cultures that normalize gathering together to eat good food or working hard as a badge of honour. So, our ways of handling stress and coping with neurodivergent symptoms can look like binge eating or workaholism. But because these coping methods are deemed as acceptable by the cultures that normalize them, we may spend our whole lives doing this without anyone realizing there's anything wrong. Rightly or wrongly, just because everyone does it, it doesn't mean that a coping method is right.

Looking at the biopsychosocial model, other factors that impact how our neurodivergence manifests include social class, religion, cognitive ability, social skills, sexual orientation and even how we look. The place we occupy in society influences the degrees of acceptance and bias we encounter, affecting the opportunities that are given to us or doors that close in our faces.

Perhaps there was a time when we intuitively knew our place, and we aspired to have everything the dominant culture had. So, we make an effort to adapt to become more like that portion of society that gets the opportunities. This can involve code switching, when someone from an underrepresented group consciously or unconsciously adjusts their natural way with spoken language, behaviour and appearance to fit into the dominant culture of that society. This goes back to our primal need to belong.

Unfortunately, it is in doing so that we find ourselves masking with several degrees of differences, leading to more internalized frustration, stress, anxiety and eventually burnout.

**Reflection**
When you took your place in society as an adult, how did the rules, norms and beliefs you internalized serve you?

## SELF-MEDICATING TO COPE WITH THE CHALLENGES OF LIFE

I've mentioned earlier how I spent a decade in existential crisis, where I would work in a job for up to a year and a half, experience burnout, quit to recover, get depressed and start again. My squiggly career is indicative of an underlying neurobiology that seeks novelty, passion and adventure – one that needed more dopamine, the molecule of reward and motivation.

A big part of what led me to seek an ADHD diagnosis was that life was really hard after I'd quit all the things that were detrimental to my mental health. I was nowhere near being fulfilled in my career and my relationship. Ironically, it made life all the more boring, slow and frankly insufferable.

For most of my twenties, I drank and partied heavily, as this was socially acceptable in my new life in England. I started drinking to help me work the room when I moved to a country that was completely different to everything I'd known.

Alcohol made me more sociable, articulate and calm. It eased my social anxiety and silenced the thoughts I had about what people were thinking about me. But while alcohol helped in the moment, the following days were terrible. It was harder to tap into focus and creativity while I was doing my PhD. It also became harder for me to maintain a consistent routine around lab work. I felt more depressed and tended to overthink.

So, when I eventually stopped my partying lifestyle, there followed periods of low moods, boredom, emptiness and loneliness that unbeknownst to me were no doubt caused by the withdrawal from the highs I'd given my brain for the last eight years. Alcohol also activates the brain centres that promote a sense of belonging, and not drinking in the company of my friends made me feel isolated.

### Vices Typical Among Neurodiverse People

Since giving talks around the country, I've discovered other things that the neurodiverse community have as their vices.

- Caffeine
- Drugs and alcohol
- Binge eating (carbs and sugar, chocolate and cakes!)
- Workaholism
- Sex and masturbating
- Relationships
- Porn
- Social media

- Playing the stockmarket
- Shopping
- Starting businesses
- Microdosing with psychedelics
- Knitting!

The trouble with constantly seeking these highs is that you're going to introduce a dopamine boost in the brain, which will undeniably be followed by a dopamine crash. The higher the high, the steeper the crash. As ADHDers, we have an inherent biology that may likely have challenges in regulating dopamine and norepinephrine homeostasis, which means some of the highs we seek can tip the balance too far that we become addicted to our vices of choice.

## Addiction and Neurodivergence

It's no wonder that so many of us have had to find ways to cope and soothe our incessant chatter in the mind. What is your own coping strategy?

This tends to be what is accepted in your culture and context and can become your 'drug of choice'. While it may include healthy sources of dopamine, such as following a nutritious diet, learning, community participation or goal attainment, it might include unhealthy sources of dopamine such as binge eating, substance use, alcohol, workaholism or relationships.

Perhaps you found ways to cope with life's challenges that are accepted in the culture you live in, so your behaviour wasn't flagged up. You may have repeated this until it became a crutch, an addiction, because you tell yourself that everyone does it. But just because everyone does it, that doesn't mean it's good for you.

If this applies to you, I'd like you to take a moment now to ask yourself what addiction might be masking for you. Perhaps there is more going on for you, besides ADHD? Perhaps you need to take the edge off life's stresses, to calm your fears, and to help you feel you can handle things on your own? Why do you think you use this coping mechanism? What support might help you?

If you're coping with an addiction problem, please seek professional evaluation and a recovery programme.

## Seeking Balance

Health is not found in the extremes. It is found in that sweet spot called balance – but how do we achieve balance, when we have an inherent biology that has challenges in regulating dopamine levels? Our habits can be rewired by replacing negative habits with positive healthy ones, as too much of anything isn't good for us.

If you don't have a serious addiction problem (and if you do, please seek medical support), Dr Anna Lembke, author of the book *Dopamine Nation*,[26] suggests the following:

**Self-binding:** physically, temporally and categorically remove the habits or people you are addicted to.
**Dopamine replacement:** replace any harmful habits with sources of 'healthy dopamine', activities that are better for you (see below for some suggestions).
**Maintaining healthy routines to increase dopamine:** these include good diet, sleep and exercise.

---

### Healthy Dopamine Activities

As for what activities constitute 'healthy dopamine', here are some of my favourite things.

- Creativity and flow state
- Mindfulness and being awestruck
- Purpose and passion

- Nutritious diet
- Breathwork and meditation
- Spending time in nature
- Being present in the here and now
- Love thyself and those around you

When you remove negative coping habits, you will gradually be able to tune in to your body and start building positive daily habits that maintain your sense of wellbeing.

## YOUR JOURNEY TO THIS POINT

When you became a young adult, you took on the world before your prefrontal cortex had fully matured, and before you were really able to make definitive decisions to support your wellbeing. This would have had an impact on the state of your nervous system and how you were around people.

You may also have needed to self-medicate so you could reliably call on your brain to do what you needed from it in every setting. However, if you consistently did so via unhealthy means, this may have compromised your brain's potential.

Now, when you look back at your life, it may be tempting to focus on any trauma you sustained in your childhood, in your life as an intersectional identity or in your current environment. The thing about masking our differences and adapting to changes on the fly, every moment of our lives leading up to now, in addition to self-medicating, has had an impact on our nervous system akin to PTSD. Trauma causes a sense of internal fragmentation, and we may struggle internally to solidify our sense of self, especially if our early beginnings didn't give us the solid foundations to make sense of our challenges, regulate our emotions, believe in ourselves, form secure partnerships with others and root our behaviours in our values. Together with the neurobiological challenges we are predisposed to, it is likely that this will manifest in mental, physical and emotional health challenges.

I hope you've adapted by developing some positive coping strategies to counteract any detrimental effects to an extent. With a bit of luck, maybe you've even found a safe person or group of people, and things have worked out for you. Perhaps your life has been potentially okay for a while, if your adaptive behaviours have served you and there are very few stressors.

But perhaps your circumstances have changed, and you now need to look after others. Maybe your loved ones rely on you. Maybe you've become a parent and found yourself responsible for another human being. Nobody ever told you that your brain and body change significantly when you become a parent, via a process known as matrescence and patrescence. You come to see the world differently, and it could be that your neurodivergent traits will come out to party, perhaps eliciting a rollercoaster of emotions.

And if you've ever found yourself in any of the situations below, you may find that your roots and routes continue to impact your resilience to deal with what life throws your way.

- Sickness, rehab or accidents
- Separation or divorce
- Grief and loss
- Menopause
- Caring for younger children or an older relative
- Discrimination incidences

Wherever your own journey through life has taken you, I hope you've had a lot of support, because every little counts. And with all the joys and adversities that life throws your way, I hope you've had people in your corner. Whatever your story, your outcome need not be dire. I am here with you now to help you make sense of the influences of nature and nurture in your life, so that you can be empowered by this knowledge and move forwards.

## UNDERSTAND YOUR LINEAGE AND MOVE FORWARD

As we've seen in this Step, you're the result of a step-by-step evolution beginning with the generations before you, through your growth in the womb and out into the world. How you manifest today as a human, your behaviours, orientations and capacities, is a result of the expression of the genes you inherited and the ones that become marked as a result of the moment-to-moment interactions in your life.

For example, as children with ADHD, many of us were told to get to an ideal endpoint without knowing how to, but this didn't help us build resilience. Instead, it created chaos inside our little brains and bodies because the neural pathways that were supposed to develop to help us process difficult thoughts and emotions hadn't become established. Instead, we learned that to be accepted we needed to play the roles society expected of us.

It's little wonder that as adults, we may deal with stress and conflicts through:

- Internalizing them
- Pushing ourselves to do more
- Panicking
- Dissociating
- Being hyper-anxious
- Slipping in passive-aggressive behaviours in disagreements

All of this affects our ability to have difficult conversations. And the way we communicate impacts the quality of our relationships. Baba Ram Dass, an American spiritual guru, said, 'In most of our human relationships, we spend much of our time reassuring one another that our costumes of identify are on straight.'[27]

Besides helping you to make sense of your behaviours, understanding your lineage shows you where there might be other factors that could render you vulnerable to certain mental and physical health conditions, so that you can make any necessary changes to your environment and lifestyle to protect yourself against them.

To understand to what extent your genes, neurotype and epigenetics have a way of shaping part of your symptoms, you could also begin by asking yourself if you're aware of any history of the following in your family:

- Neurodevelopmental conditions
- Mental health conditions
- Chronic health conditions
- Long-term physical health issues
- Self-medicating tendencies and the outcome of the family member involved

## Genetic Testing

If you want to go further to understand any potential genetic predispositions you might have to certain conditions, you could order a genetic test for yourself. While having the genes may not necessarily mean you're going to manifest these conditions, it does mean that what you choose to do every day will either increase or decrease your chances of developing them.

To address your specific needs, you need to be aware of the following things.

1. The presence of co-occurring mental and physical health conditions.
2. Contributing factors that can increase risk, such as sleep quality, stress, diet, alcohol, drugs, and sensory, hormonal and relationship challenges.
3. When and how you're potentially vulnerable to challenges when contributing factors are at play, causing for example reduced executive function, emotional challenges or a tendency to be impulsive.
4. Lifestyle changes and clinical support needed for your mental and physical needs.

With this knowledge, it's important to create a prevention programme as outlined in Step 2 to avoid the worst-case scenarios.

As there are so many interconnected factors at play in our neurodivergence, support needs to be addressed on an individual basis and via a holistic lens, which ideally includes coordinated efforts from multi-disciplinary teams that can recommend strategies informed from a combination of lived experience, science, clinical research, psychiatric observations and lifestyle alterations.

You can also play an important part in this process yourself by identifying your potential vulnerabilities and recognizing your patterns of behaviour so that you can modify them in ways that will support your physical and mental wellbeing.

### Recognize Your Everyday Patterns of Behaviour

Behaviour is a form of communication. I first heard this said to describe the behaviours we see in neurodivergent kids who struggle with internal challenges without the words to explain why. This gave me more compassion for the things my kids say to me, especially in the midst of a meltdown. It also opened my eyes to what was happening to us late-diagnosed adults with ADHD who are going back to our workplaces and telling our managers and colleagues about our neurodivergence, and opening up about it at home. In an effort to be true to ourselves, many of us are finding that the only way to be authentic is to own our neurodivergence.

The challenge with this is that while we may be mentally ready, our emotions, nervous system and body aren't ready. So these conversations don't always go well. As we've seen, our emotional capacities and nervous systems have not been given the chance to mature. We are all little kids playing adults. Perhaps if we have a heightened stress response, then we're very likely to get triggered when we encounter familiar triggers in our daily life. These patterns of behaviour have a way of replaying until we resolve them.

The first step towards showing up as a better version of ourselves is to observe our own behaviours and notice how we are showing up, so we can learn to show up better.

1. **Get to know yourself:** Pay attention to how you act and react in different situations. See how you usually respond to different triggers and events.
2. **Regularly journal about your thoughts, feelings and actions:** This can help you see any repeating patterns in your interactions at home, work or social settings over time.
3. **Ask for advice:** Talk to people you trust – family or friends – about how they see your behaviour. They might notice things that you haven't.
4. **Think back on past experiences:** Recall times when you felt a certain way or behaved in a particular manner. Try to find common themes or reactions in those moments.
5. **Be aware of changing circumstances:** These might concern the following:
   - Biological changes
   - Stress management
   - Sleep
   - Nutrition
   - Executive functioning
   - Emotional regulation
   - Emotional and mental processing speed
   - Trauma from growing up with undiagnosed neurodivergence or trauma from being an intersectional identity
   - Relational trauma
6. **Seek help from a therapist or counsellor:** This may be a professional that can help you make sense of these behaviour patterns, help you explore your emotions in a safe space, and guide you towards understanding and potentially changing them.

Plenty of love and light to you as you dissect your life and the adaptive behaviours you acquired, and learn to reframe your experiences to see how these overlap with those of others. There are certain experiences we share as a neurodivergent community that are shaped by our gender, being part of a global majority or person of colour, or having grown up in a certain social class, which can throw life out of whack for us. Because frankly, no one is untouched by life.

# Step 5:
# Identify Your Emotional Needs

When I use biology to explain neurodivergent behaviours and destigmatize ADHD and autism, I always get comments back from a neurodivergent audience who feel validated for their ways of being. Perhaps there is a very big part of us that feels comforted that biology has a big role in determining our behaviour; it lessens the pain we've endured from what we couldn't control.

In every setting where I give a talk, whenever I ask a group of ADHDers, 'What's your deepest fear as a neurodivergent?' the answer is always unanimously this: to be misunderstood.

It can be really hard to explain to someone that you're living with an invisible neurodevelopmental condition that affects your entire being, not just the brain. Sometimes, we may feel completely at a loss as to what to do when we see how our involuntary actions can result in undesired consequences in the relationships and interactions in our lives, leaving us to feel ostracized by the very unit or community we live in.

In Step 5 of the ADHD iceberg, we are going to look at how we can sometimes struggle in relationships and the brain differences that may lie behind this. We'll also consider what happens when things really go wrong, and the complications of trauma and post-traumatic stress disorder (PTSD). Finally, I will be sharing some strategies to help you identify your emotional needs and manage your life in supportive ways that will enable you to regulate yourself emotionally.

## STANDING OUT FROM THE CROWD

It certainly takes a lot of courage to stand out from the crowd. But maybe it's not so hard if your inherent authentic way of being means it's incredibly hard to be anything other than you?

I can still see her now, the little girl who went through life trying so hard to give people what they needed from her in every situation she found herself in. Sometimes, it would feel really difficult to summon up the energy for social interactions. Why wouldn't her brain and body switch on when she needs them?

And at times she would use food, sugar and fizzy drinks to give her the energy to engage with the world. When all she really wanted was to be in a state of flow, single-mindedly creating, crafting and daydreaming. In school, she had friends who were just like her, so it was okay for a while. And when she did overstep the mark with them, they didn't always tell her.

As she grew into a young adult and began university, she realized that her natural ways weren't enough anymore. There were more social and societal expectations for her to be more pleasing, humble, selfless and to think more of others. But she carried on being herself for a while, someone who loves to learn and share what she knows, someone who is honest to a fault, someone who frankly prefers books to human interactions.

She could be bluntly honest, and this, she learned from feedback, is socially unacceptable. She was misunderstood, gossiped about and bullied. 'When people don't understand who you are, they make up their own stories about you,' is what one of her bullies told her when she opened up to them. She learned that not everyone is nice, and that people seem to bring their own histories into relationships, and project their wounds onto one another.

She learned to adapt, she learned to mask. She learned to be everything that she wasn't by mimicking others who were more sociable. She felt like she was the only person who didn't receive the memo for how to do this. And it started to work and people started to like her.

But she had to double-down on concealing the real person within, to share more of the parts that other people liked, so she felt she belonged.

It still doesn't always work. Her emotions can flare from zero to a hundred when she encounters a trigger, followed by shame and guilt after the feelings have subsided. And these triggers are often violations of her sense of autonomy, to be able to do things her way. It seems to be impossible to control the tsunami of feelings and thoughts that flood her mind, as they're nearly always beyond her control. Emotions have ruled her life, and she always attempts to repair any damage done by over-explaining and then blaming herself.

How can she ever hope to be true to herself, if deep down she doesn't even know what she is made of? Without a stable anchor, she is like a feather, blown into the direction the wind chooses to go. Filling the air of every space she encounters.

But she does have a compass. One that is buried so deep, and now she has found her way to connect with it. And she aims to show you this too.

Because at the end of the day, I think we can all agree that we want to be us. To be us is the best so far. Because it's such a rarity to be loved for us, to be understood and accepted, to be validated and seen for our challenges, but not singled out as different. To belong because we are authentically ourselves.

We just need to get comfortable asking for what we need.

## WHEN OUR NEEDS AREN'T UNDERSTOOD

One of the biggest revelations I've had from working with adults in the field of neurodiversity is seeing the many ways in which we can manifest our unmet emotional needs. On the surface, this can look like any of the following:

- Fight (externalizing our emotions), flight (internalizing our emotions, avoiding communication), fawn (such as people-pleasing behaviours), freeze (dissociation), fib (lying), faint (temporary loss of consciousness).

- States of emotional hyper-arousal or hypo-arousal, such as meltdown or shutdown from sensory overwhelm.
- Hyper-empathy or hypo-empathy that can trigger misunderstandings.
- Rejection sensitivity dysphoria (RSD), with symptoms such as intense sadness, shame or anger after perceived rejection, or heightened fear of abandonment or criticism.
- Emotional and mental distress during life transitions.
- Psychological stress and its catastrophic impact.
- Eagerness to repair from shame and guilt, rather than from an authentic place of wanting to make amends.
- Self-abandonment.
- Co-dependency.
- Unsteady sense of self.
- Chronic overwhelm from taking on more than we can manage and not asking for help and/or burnout (physically, mentally or emotionally).
- The empath-narcissist or anxious-avoidant partner combination (see Step 6, page 189).

By the time neurodivergents show these behaviours, our nervous systems and bodies are already on the defensive. The activation of our sympathetic nervous system, decrease in serotonin and oxytocin, spikes in cortisol from relational and other life stresses, and the full repertoire of the stress response may cause us to appear reactive or conflict-avoidant, to be people-pleasing, to mask, and to struggle with anxiety and depression. While experiencing the emotional turbulence of all of this, we may lack an understanding of our own internal experience, let alone the words to talk about it. This is why being understood is so important, and is the loudest way to say 'I see you'.

While we, as ADHDers, may tend to associate emotions with fleeting responses to events and people, these surface presentations have deeper biological roots.

## THE WAY WE'RE EMOTIONALLY WIRED

I love this quote from the Hindu scripture the Bhagavad Gita: 'We never really encounter the world, all we ever experience is our own nervous system.' All day long, our nervous systems decide how we feel about the people and places we come across, and events that take place.

Have you stopped to think about what this system looks like? What are emotions and behaviours from a biological perspective, and what regulates them? The human nervous system is divided into two branches, the central nervous system composed of the brain and spine, and the peripheral nervous system composed of the somatic and autonomous nervous systems.

Think of your brain as being like a symphony orchestra made up of different sections (such as strings, brass and percussion). Each section has its own speciality, but they have to play in harmony for everything to sound right.

**The Conductor:** prefrontal cortex (decision-making, planning, impulse control)
**Emotion section:** limbic system (especially the amygdala and hippocampus, handles emotion and memory)
**Survival percussion:** brain stem and hypothalamus (basic bodily functions and threat detection)
**Communication and balance sections:** cerebellum and brain networks (coordinate movement, social cues, sensory processing)

### How the Neurodivergent Nervous System is Different From the Neurotypical

Quite simply, we are born to feel, see and hear more. And our conductor (the prefrontal cortex) sometimes shows up late – or gets drowned out by the drums.

As we saw in Step 3, autistic individuals begin life on a different neurodevelopmental baseline. We experience a period of rapid brain development where the volume of the amygdala increases greatly from six to twelve months. Early in life, there are patterns of atypical local connectivity in autistic brain regions, both via hyper-connectivity (unusually dense growth of neurons and their firing in five brain networks – the salience, default mode, frontotemporal, moto, and visual networks) and hypo-connectivity (unusually sparse growth of neurons and their firing and disruptions in long-range connectivity between left parietal and temporal lobes and in the right frontal and temporal regions.)[1]

The salience network, which integrates information about sensory, emotional and cognitive information, is the most heavily hyper-connected network in autism. Autistic individuals also may have altered empathetic pain-related skin conductor response. When we are exposed to pain experienced by other people, we can have higher levels of physical and sympathetic nervous system activation. Not being able to recognize or detect these signals accurately comes at a cost – the anxiety can mount and we feel emotions more intensely.

ADHDers also have differences in brain structure sizes, volume and connectivity. The size of the amygdala, hippocampus and cerebellum are thought to be atypical, with imbalances in dopamine and norepinephrine levels in the prefrontal cortex, amygdala, basal ganglia and the reticular activating system. As we saw in Step 2, the development of the prefrontal cortex, the brain control centre, is delayed for two to five years compared to our peers, and has been thought to not fully mature in the ADHD brain until at least 35 years of age. The bottom-up signalling (taking sensory information and processing it) is also stronger than the top-down signalling (using pre-existing knowledge and thinking to guide behaviour).

## THE IMPLICATIONS OF BRAIN STRUCTURAL DIFFERENCES ON ADHDERS' EMOTIONS

- We take on more sensory inputs from the world, and can struggle to integrate or make sense of them.
- We have an absolute desperation to avoid boredom and routine.

- We have an increased tendency to ruminate, and challenges in regulating emotions.
- We face challenges to inhibit impulsive and unwanted behaviours.
- We persistently pull away from what we are trying to focus on if it doesn't hold our interest.
- We show increased novelty-seeking and sensation-seeking.
- We can be more feeling, rather than thinking, beings and we always rely on our instincts even in the midst of decision paralysis.

Autistic individuals and ADHDers are also thought to have less effective communication between the prefrontal cortex (brain control centre) and our emotional brain (the limbic centre). This can manifest as emotional flooding or an intense emotional experience, with challenges in tapping into the rational brain to process emotions in the moment or think about long-term consequences.

Meanwhile, for those of us who are AuDHDers, researchers found distinctive brain dynamics characterized by patterns of socio-communication found in those with pure autism spectrum disorder (ASD), but with an unstable neural activity of the prefrontal area that triggers a whole-brain over-flexible activity, which is different to that seen in pure ADHD.[2] The significance of this means that as AuDHDers, we are more likely to possess brain dynamics that are prone to both inflexibility and chaos.

With growing curiosity around the mysteries of neurodivergent proficiency (or lack thereof) in emotional regulation, many in the neurodiverse community have become experts themselves around nervous system regulation in relation to the autonomic nervous system (ANS). This can be further divided into two branches: the sympathetic nervous system (SNS) and the parasympathetic nervous system (PNS).

Our ANS holds the key to understanding our emotional needs, and the reason it has received so much airtime is due to our fight-or-flight or 'mobilization' response that often underlies the 'zero to a hundred' emotional dysregulation seen in autistic people and ADHDers.

Today, in our daily lives, we don't often get into combative mode right away or flee out the door when we are triggered. More often, though, our response to emotional and social triggers is to dissociate or avoid (freeze), people-please (fawn), lie (fib), or in more extreme circumstances that overwhelm our senses, we may indeed faint or shutdown.

On the surface, it may look like the ADHDer you have started a new relationship with suddenly withdraws within themselves after a disagreement, or your co-worker who started off really enthusiastic and agreeable has now gone quieter, or you may sense that your sweet daughter suddenly learns to lie about something she knew she would get in trouble about.

These may seem like normal reactions to stressful daily situations which everyone may go through, but for a neurodivergent individual, these situations may be the final stressor that tips a nervous system in survival mode over the edge.

Have you ever thought about what creates these intense emotional responses in many neurodivergents? It often happens so quickly and involuntarily that it's hard to imagine a higher power at work in our brain.

That's because it is often unconscious, involuntary and *automatic*.

## POLYVAGAL THEORY

The polyvagal theory, introduced in 1994 by Dr Stephen Porges, offers three core ideas that I believe are foundational to our understanding of the nervous system.

1. **The autonomic hierarchy:** the ANS is divided into two circuits (SNS and PNS) and three pre-set pathways that have physical, emotional and mental effects in the body. They are:
    - Ventral vagal: the system of connection (supports feelings of safety, social connection and calm)
    - Sympathetic: the system of action (mobilizes energy for survival)

- Dorsal vagal: the system of shutdown (triggers immobilization or collapse when a situation feels overwhelming, leading to numbness, disconnection or freeze states)
2. **Neuroception:** a built-in system in the body that scans our internal and external environments for signs of safety or danger and activates appropriate neural circuits.
3. **Co-regulation:** the subconscious action of syncing up with others with a coherent nervous system who have the strongest safety cue to facilitate wellbeing.

In Step 3, we looked briefly at the vagus nerve in relation to vagal tone, which is lower in ADHDers. The vagus nerve, known as the wandering nerve, is the longest cranial nerve and starts at the brain stem and branches into the face, connecting to multiple sensory organs and vital organs, which include the heart, lungs, stomach, intestines, pancreas and more. It plays an important role in activating the parasympathetic branch of the nervous system through ventral and dorsal vagal activation. Despite its name, the vagus nerve isn't a single nerve, but a bundle of nerves that connects the body and brain through a two-way communication, with 80 per cent of the information going from the body to the brain, and 20 per cent from the brain to the body. Porges hypothesizes that faulty neuroception can contribute to psychiatric conditions, as some brains are biased towards detecting danger when there is no real danger.

Rather than possessing a faulty neuroception, as we have seen, we begin life on a different baseline, and it is from here that we have to make sense of the world we live in. In Step 3, we touched on how autistic individuals and ADHDers are born with innate physical and sensory sensitivities that can bestow us with a lower threshold for handling external stressors and it is from there that our nervous system goes into the world. Add to this our neurodevelopmental differences and, as we saw in Step 4, the imprinting of attachment issues from our significant relationships early in life through to the present.

Perhaps we all have an early memory of knowing we are different to others. For me, this was when I stood in a queue wearing nothing but a white singlet and underwear in kindergarten. I had got wet playing in the rain because I hadn't heard the teacher call us into the classroom when it started raining hard. I was soaked, and there were no other decent clothes for me to change into. While this seems like an innocent event, to me it was confusing: why hadn't I heard the teacher call us in? To my knowledge, I didn't have a hearing problem. But I always seemed to end up in embarrassing or alarming situations because I'd missed the memo, whether this was due to not hearing verbal instructions or not being able to process them in a way that allowed me to take the appropriate action.

There would be many more incidents in different circumstances throughout primary school that continued to confuse me until, finally, in secondary school, when the things that helped me cope (such as athletics and physical exercise) were no longer part of my daily routine and I began to experience hormonal changes, my differences created significant challenges. I knew I had to do something about it.

This was also when I began to feel nervous in every new situation, adapting rapidly to meet other people's expectations or hiding away from others so I wouldn't be singled out for what I thought were character flaws. Over time, my adaptive strategies made me so far removed from who I believed I really was that it was difficult to know what was right or wrong anymore. It felt like I was always in survival mode, and the only way to get out of it was to channel my thoughts into what I thought was positive, to achieve academically. Because when I was engaged in learning, not only was I in a flow state which was so rewarding in itself, but the praise I got from achieving good grades made me feel worthy.

So what happens when we push a neurodivergent's nervous system too far, without much support at all?

## THE ADHD BODY IN SURVIVAL MODE

James Ochoa, author of *Focused Forward: Navigating the Storms of Adult ADHD*,[3] claims that the effects that lifelong ADHD-related stress can have on our nervous system can be likened to post-traumatic stress disorder (PTSD). He calls this emotional distress syndrome, a cumulative effect of brain-processing differences and behavioural changes associated with ADHD which wears down our emotional tolerance, stamina and sense of wellbeing.

In fact, a systematic review showed that there is indeed a bi-directional relationship between ADHD and PTSD, whereby:

- ADHDers are four times more likely to be at risk of PTSD than those without ADHD.
- Those who suffer with PTSD are twice as likely to also have ADHD.[4]

Similarly, studies show that autistic individuals are up to 60 per cent more likely to experience PTSD, and it is believed that the characteristics of ASD can affect what is perceived as trauma.[5] Autistic individuals reported a broad range of life events as traumatic, including:

- Traumas classified as such within DSM-5 (the *Diagnostic and Statistical Manual of Mental Disorders*) – sexual and physical abuse
- Non-DSM-5 traumas – bullying, bereavement and traumas related to mental health problems such as 'breakdowns'
- Novel non-DSM-5 traumas – the ASD diagnostic process, experience of therapy, being disturbed by one's violence towards others, and unannounced visits from the police

Despite many studies suggesting autistic individuals have a heightened sympathetic activation and lower resilience to stress, a recent study refuted this widely accepted belief, at least in autistic children.[6] They found that the data from almost all studies on heart rate variability (HRV) in autistic kids, which measures (ANS) nervous system activity, show that there is no evidence of general autonomic dysfunction associated with typical ASD traits, despite studies concluding the opposite. However, some autistic kids do have a reaction to stimuli that falls outside what's considered the 'normal range', with relatively high heart rate associated with autonomic dysfunction such as anxiety or gastrointestinal dysfunctions.

Perhaps not everyone with ADHD or ASD is born with heightened emotional volatility; rather, being born with an innate sensitivity to the world leads us to perceive certain experiences as more stressful than other people. When they say ADHDers and autistic individuals tend to have a less flexible and adaptable nervous system, this is likely a result of our needing to adapt to an unpredictable, ever-changing world that is often not made for our brain differences, often while having trouble switching gears.

Within the neurodiverse community, the spectrum of our emotional experiences can range from those who are able to access resources to get to a more regulated mental state, those who are out of touch with their emotions and perhaps struggle to explain their range of emotions, and those who struggle with mental disorders.

If we go back to the science of safety, we can almost see the development of a nervous system whose window of tolerance has very varied bandwidths. (The 'window of tolerance', or rather the 'window of capacity', is where we are able to function effectively. It is the optimal emotional zone for us to thrive in, as defined by professor of psychiatry Dan Siegel; see Step 5, page 164, and Step 9, page 278, for more on this helpful concept). So what creates the differences between a healthy nervous system that is able to switch back relatively quickly to the ventral vagal state of calm, safety and social engagement (also known as connection mode), versus one that is stuck in dorsal vagal or sympathetic activation, also known as survival mode?

Perhaps we may see 'survival mode' more commonly in those who have been subjected to early experiences that activate the fear centre in the brain, as discussed earlier. A study by Joseph Biederman and colleagues found a deficient fear circuitry in young adult ADHDers when compared to those without ADHD.[7] The fear circuit consists of different brain areas which interact with each other during distinct phases:

1. **Fear acquisition:** when the brain perceives that one is in danger.
2. **Extinction learning:** the brain 'cools' and learns to stop being afraid of something that it used to associate with danger or harm even though the danger was no longer there.
3. **Consolidation of the learning:** lessons learned from the experience.
4. **Extinction of fear memory recall:** the memory associated with fear is extinguished.

Using functional magnetic resonance (fMRI) imaging, they found that ADHDers show less activity in the ventromedial prefrontal cortex, hippocampus, dorsal anterior cingulate cortex and insula activation, which are involved in fear extinction learning and extinction memory, or learning to overcome fear.

While both ADHDers and individuals with PTSD show similar brain deficiencies when it comes to remembering how to let go of fear, ADHDers seemed to remember better when tested the next day. This suggests that while ADHDers might struggle to create new memories of safety in the same situations where the fear was learned, they are better at finding new ways to manage and reduce past fears.

When we hold on to the fear of what's happened to us – or even what's happened *within* us – our brains do something pretty clever. They adapt, often in ways that help protect us from having to relive those painful experiences all over again.

But that protection can come with a cost. It might show up as:

- Feeling emotionally numb or carrying invisible wounds.
- Developing coping strategies that help in the moment, but might not serve us long-term.
- Being constantly on edge – always scanning for danger (hello, hyper-vigilance).
- Or checking out completely when things get too much (what we call dissociation).

The thing is, that fear doesn't disappear. It gets buried deep inside, quietly waiting for the next trigger to pull it back to the surface.

Now, let's not forget that the prefrontal cortex of ADHDers may not fully mature until the age of 35 or 40. So that creates a pretty big window for us to encounter many experiences that we may perceive as threatening, and for our fear-anxiety circuit to activate our fear responses before our rational brain fully matures. As you can see, this means that we're always one step behind in terms of processing how we feel about our lives, as they unfold before our eyes.

Is it any wonder that repeated cycles of stress can kickstart a fear-fight-flight-anxiety/depression-freeze-fawn-or-fib maladaptive response? Rather than us being born with an innate heightened nervous system, it is plausible that this repeated exposure to worldly stressors, combined with physical vulnerabilities, is what causes our ANS dysregulation. Our nervous system flips from a state of hyper-arousal (sympathetic mode) to hypo-arousal (dorsal mode), and vice versa. Our body may also struggle with HPA axis dysfunction, producing imbalanced levels of the stress hormones cortisol and adrenaline for prolonged periods and leaving us less resilient to stress.

As emotional expressions are a language of social interactions, how we express ourselves is a learned response from the interactions and relationships we have within our homes and place in society.

## THE ROOT OF OUR PAIN AND HOW WE SHOW UP

My exploration into the question of whether our reactions are because of ADHD or trauma began when I looked into the number of neurodivergents who have had adverse childhood experiences (ACEs), whether in the form of physical, emotional, mental or sexual abuse in their lives. In nearly every talk I gave, people told me that they felt truly seen for the first time when I talked about what happens within us when we encounter situations in our daily lives that activate the traumatic imprint that has lain dormant for decades in our bodies.

The thing about trauma is that all trauma practitioners agree that it isn't what happened *to* you, but rather what happened *within* you. Trauma occurs during moments in life when you're faced with situations that your nervous system deems are dangerous, and you have to figure out what to do very quickly without any support from someone you trust to guide you into safety.

To be clear, I'm not saying that all neurodivergents have had trauma in their lives, or that all neurodivergents who have experienced trauma will continue to live in a state of autonomic dysfunction. But that the picture is complex.

As neurodivergent adults, when our emotional systems become hijacked, it can be difficult to regulate our emotions. Some emotions may lead us to lose the joy of living, while other emotions may lead us to seek reward and develop addictive tendencies. To begin to understand this, we need to look into our emotional systems, which originate from the primal survival instincts we inherited from our mammalian evolutionary ancestors.

According to Jaak Panksepp, an Estonian-American neuroscientist who studied the neural mechanisms of emotions, there are at least seven primary emotion systems. These are biologically inherited and are responsible for our core emotional patterns; they are concentrated in the subcortical regions of all mammalian brains.[8]

These emotional systems are initially activated by unconditional stimuli, which trigger a reflexive and instinctive behaviour. Once aroused, our emotions can outlast the event that caused them in the first place. Our emotional systems also regulate many sensory inputs into the brain and, therefore, control learning and programme higher brain cognitive abilities. Our emotions are then regulated by higher brain processes when the brain matures.

As discussed in Steps 3 and 4, we neurodivergents have neurodevelopmental differences that may predispose us to different ways of forming social connections, processing information, reacting to sensory cues, seeking rewards and regulating our distress. From birth, we're wired to seek attachment and emotional connection with our caregivers to develop our nervous systems. If we were attuned to

## The Seven Primary Emotion Systems

| EMOTION SYSTEM | EMOTIONAL PATTERN |
|---|---|
| CARE (maternal nurturance system) | The urge for parents to nurture and protect their children. When aroused among adult partners it may promote a satisfying relationship. |
| LUST (sexual system) | Aroused by male and female sexual hormones, which control many brain chemistries, including social neuropeptides such as oxytocin (promoted by oestrogen in females) and vasopressin (promoted by testosterone in males). Activities can also be driven by the dopamine-driven SEEKING system in search of sexual rewards. |
| PLAY (physical social engagement system) | The key function of social play is to learn social rules and refine social interactions. PLAY may promote empathy and activate the neurochemistry that's useful in treating depression. |
| SEEKING (desire system) | The 'brain reward and motivational system', a major source of life 'energy'. In its pure form, this provokes intense and enthusiastic exploration and anticipatory excitement/ learning in all types of reward. |
| RAGE (anger system) | Provoked when we lose freedom in our actions. It lies close to and interacts with FEAR systems – likely an implicit source of the 'fight-or-flight' response. |
| FEAR (anxiety system) | Protects us from pain and destruction. People with an activated FEAR system are overcome by an intense free-floating anxiety that appears to have no external causes. |
| GRIEF, formerly known as PANIC (separation distress system) | Helps us stay connected to others we depend on. When GRIEF is activated – during loss, disconnection or abandonment – it can trigger deep sadness, longing and a sense of emotional pain. |

them, responded to emotionally, and have at least one sane parent who we can turn to whatever the situation, and who accepts us just as we are, we're more likely to have a wider window of tolerance.

The emotional world of neurodivergent children can be an intense, all-or-nothing experience. If you consider the fact that we can often feel unprepared for the world with its pace, volume, brightness, temperature and demands, it's not surprising that we may lean towards an avoidant or anxious disposition that colours our personality and emotional response. We can be under-stimulated or overstimulated, sensory-seeking or sensory-avoidant, depending on our contexts.

Many parents of neurodivergents could be neurodivergents themselves, with their own issues. Even with the best of intentions, parenting a child with sensory and emotional needs can trigger your own experiences of how you were parented, and therefore activate the unique traumatic imprints on your nervous system from your own childhood. In daily parenting, without knowing about the brain differences around executive function, socio-communication or emotional regulation, the behaviours of children with ADHD can often confuse their parents in turn. All this can manifest in an unpredictable household, one where one or both of our parents swing towards the extreme end of parenting approaches, being over-controlling or too relaxed (to the point of neglect) and life can be a rollercoaster ride.

Moreover, every culture has its norms, whether that's allowing babies to cry so they can learn to soothe themselves, or rewarding and punishing behaviours that are considered 'good' or 'bad'. However, these strategies don't always work on neurodivergents with an interest-based nervous system or a persistent drive for autonomy; instead, they place demands on us to respond in ways that aren't authentic or true to what we want. It doesn't activate our intrinsic motivation. For example, inconsistent parenting strategies, such as agreeing to give a reward and then retracting it in order to discipline a child, essentially using the proffered reward as a punishment instead, don't give a child a stable and safe foundation on which to base their own value judgements and can activate their SEEKING, FEAR, GRIEF and RAGE systems.

Living in the world with a neurodevelopmental difference can feel confusing. It's a bit like turning up to a party and not adhering to the right dress code. We can find ourselves saying 'unusual' or socially inappropriate things that can make us seem weird and make us vulnerable to the bullying behaviours of others. We might often miss chunks of conversations. Walk around with our shoelaces undone or drive with our coats trapped in the doors of our cars. It can mean forgetting where we put our keys and locking ourselves out of the house. It's like we're constantly under-equipped to deal with what the world throws our way. Unless we become inflexible and perfectionistic, there is always a sense that we've forgotten to do something.

One of my biggest challenges as an AuDHDer to date is in understanding people's intentions, emotions and thoughts. When I am unclear about somebody's intentions, this can provoke an intense FEAR/anxiety response within me, and I will react by avoiding any demands made on me.

Imagine going into the world like this, scrambling to adapt, finding ways to cope, and finally feeling like you can relax. Then the need for novelty rears its head and you end up diving into a new situation before you are prepared to deal with it.

As touched upon in Step 3, many of our challenges tend to become more apparent during distinct periods of change or major life transitions in which our environments change before we've developed the strategies to deal with them. The unpredictability of events that occur beyond our control can lead to emotional distress such as depression, which researchers believe is due to diminished CARE and PLAY, and elevated FEAR and RAGE brain networks. Depression can feel unusually bad and painful from over-activity of the GRIEF network that sends an individual into chronic despair, promoting abnormally low reward-SEEKING behaviour.[9]

To paraphrase Bessel van der Kolk, author of *The Body Keeps the Score*,[10] trauma disrupts the inner barometer of what we feel; that is, it impairs our ability to trust our gut feelings. It's the sign of a system pushed too far in survival response, one that doesn't feel safe in its own body.

## THE RISKS OF SUPPRESSING OUR NEEDS

Over time, we learn that the only way to be loved – to have a 'healthy attachment' to others – and to belong, is to do what other people want us to do. Which may mean masking our own authentic emotional needs. As Gabor Maté, author of *The Myth of Normal*,[11] says, children may forgo authenticity to seek attachment with their caregivers. We then wrestle with these two needs: to belong or to be authentic?

If we grew up in a household where our parents were always stressed, under-resourced or couldn't support our emotions, then we are likely to have repressed our emotions and never learned that we needed to attach and support the development of our emotional systems in a healthy manner.

Children who have been emotionally neglected may grow up to become adults whose emotional states can swing from one extreme of being hyper-vigilant (anxious) to another extreme of being dissociative (avoidant or depressed) when they encounter stressors. This can look like:

**Disconnection from our own emotions:** we have difficulty explaining upset, anger or excitement, or regulating our emotions, leading to meltdown or shutdown.
**Doubling down:** making more effort, bordering on perfectionism to seek external validation.
**Defensive behaviours:** not saying sorry or owning a mistake even when it's our fault. This is likely because we've grown used to needing to defend ourselves, being told we are too much or being ignored until we calm down.
**Hyper-independence:** not knowing how to ask for help or believing we need help.
**People-pleasing:** doing things to ensure other people are okay first so we will be okay, not being able to voice our needs, overpromising.
**Shame:** the smallest mistake can induce the biggest shame.

**Escapism:** always looking for an exit point so we can be alone as we may find it overwhelming being around people.
**Compulsive lying:** feeling it's unsafe to tell the truth and guarding one's personal truth as one's safe space instead.
**Decision paralysis:** finding it hard to make decisions; if we're not connected to our emotions, it can be hard to know how we feel. This can feel like being frozen because in the past it was deemed unacceptable for us to exert an opinion.
**Looking for emotionally unavailable partners:** this lack of connection is familiar and paradoxically comforting to one's nervous system.

The reality is that the trauma of growing up with a neurodevelopmental difference, when compounded by intersectional experiences such as gender, social class, race or ethnicity, can create additional complexities in our path to recovery.

Now imagine how trauma takes hold on our psyche over time and how it feels within our body. It is unsurprising that:

- Certain interactions and relationships trigger an emotional response that is of a larger magnitude than warranted.
- Neurodivergents can struggle with mental ill health due to emotional dysregulation.
- Intersectional neurodivergents can manifest trauma in their body as high blood pressure or chest pain instead of having the vocabulary to express their emotions.

## RECOGNIZE YOUR REALITY

Whenever I mentor neurodivergents, I always ask them questions that will help them clarify what their needs are in their present realities, such as 'Where in your life are you feeling most supported – or not?' and, 'What's one thing you wish others would understand about your needs right now?' Even if we are all on a similar journey of moving ahead following an understanding of our neurotype, our neurodiverse experiences vary greatly.

When I talk about the realities of being a neurodivergent woman, it's from a place of really wanting to be understood myself. I often get comments from other neurodivergents who say we're all neurodivergent, so can we try to avoid dividing up the label? But our behaviour is an expression of our emotional state, which, as we've seen, is based on our internal biological, psychological state, and our nervous system. Our worldly experiences and interactions that we encounter at different ages and stages all have an impact on our emotional states. Without talking about how our reality contributes to the diversity in our neurodiverse experiences, how are we going to get to the bottom of what our unique needs are?

As we have seen, within the neurodiverse community, our emotional needs vary based on compounding differences such as:

- The genes we inherit
- Impact on gene expression from environmental stimuli
- Our history, including the presence of ACEs, PTSD or complex post-traumatic stress disorder (CPTSD)
- Protective childhood experiences that counter ACEs and build our resilience
- Gender
- Age
- Socio-economic factors
- History of substance use disorder
- Traumatic life transitions
- Joys in life
- Current caring responsibilities
- Current support network
- Quality of significant relationships
- Adherence to sensory, physical, emotional, mental and social self-care needs
- Level of stressors at our stage of life

Whoever we are, our internal world is in a constant state of flux and both innate and external factors affect our ability to feel a sense of emotional safety within. For example, knowing that our identity and life circumstance add degrees of complexities to how we show up can help prevent the misunderstanding we seem to find ourselves in.

## WIDEN YOUR WINDOW OF TOLERANCE

Our window of tolerance is a state in which we feel calm, connected and engaged, and relates to the ventral vagal and social engagement systems (see page 150). In a balanced autonomic state, our sympathetic and parasympathetic states are able to perform their regulating roles, while our ventral energy oversees the system.

Many neurodivergents have a narrower window of tolerance due to a combination of factors in their neurology, biology, psychology and sociology, and life's stressors can kick us out our window of tolerance into hyper-arousal (sympathetic activation), or hypo-arousal (parasympathetic immobilization).

Regulating our emotions involves learning the skills to widen our window of tolerance, so we can come out of a hyper-aroused or hypo-aroused state more easily. (For more on this, see Step 9, page 278.)

---

### Master Your Emotions

To widen your own window of tolerance, you will need to develop an awareness of how you're showing up in the present to reach emotional regulation. You can learn how to do this by using the following steps.

1. Tune in to your internal state and notice how your body feels: where are you in terms of your emotional state?

2. Are you hyper-aroused or hypo-aroused? In other words, do you feel overcome by emotion or drained of it?
3. If you feel heightened emotions such as anxiety or upset, you can employ distress tolerance tools, including self-regulating tools such as breathwork, meditation, yoga, Pilates or taking warm baths or cold showers – whatever works best for you.
4. Try to co-regulate with a safe person or pet.
5. Anchor yourself in safety and regulation, perhaps by thinking of someone you trust, connecting with your body through simple stretches, or listening to calming music. Once you have identified your triggers, you can turn to these sorts of simple practices as a way to bring yourself back into balance.

Other long-term strategies you can explore to support your nervous system include:

- Processing and releasing emotional wounds and traumas through compassion-focused therapy or psychedelic-assisted therapy
- Eye Movement Desensitization and Reprocessing (EMDR)
- Dialectical Behavioural Therapy (DBT)
- Acceptance and Commitment Therapy (ACT)
- Somatic therapy
- Mindfulness meditation
- Ensuring adequate sleep, diet and exercise, managing inflammation and detoxification
- Being aware of your triggers – the things that cause you to experience strong emotions or to behave in certain ways – and being mindful to avoid or address them

## SENSORY OVERWHELM

The nature of being a neurodivergent is that our hyper-sensitivity to sensory stimuli can create an automatic emotional response in our nervous system which happens so quickly it feels as though we don't have any say in the matter.

Sensory overwhelm can creep up on ADHDers and autistic individuals because it can be difficult to sense what's happening internally – until a tidal wave of meltdown crashes onto the shore, leaving a scene of destruction that brings upon more trauma than we bargained for. So, our capacity to show up in the world relies on us doing the one thing that we are also terrible at doing – being aware of our energy levels.

### Do Your Own Energy Accounting

Dr Tony Attwood, a world-renowned clinical psychologist and expert on autism, developed an energy accounting tool with Maja Toudal. It encourages us to think of our energy like a bank account and how every task, interaction or sensory exposure either withdraws from or deposits into that account. It is incredibly helpful to help us identify what activities in our daily lives are giving us energy and which are depleting it so we know where we are in our energy tanks.

The idea is to compile a list of things that recharge your battery and a list of things that use up your energy, then give them each a score in terms of the intensity you feel each activity gives or takes your energy. When numerous withdrawals have been made, deposits need to be made in order to avoid going into energy deficit or meltdown.

To receive the full benefits of energy accounting, I would suggest that you visit the Energy Accounting website.[12] In the meantime, here are a couple of simple steps to get you started:

## STEP 5: IDENTIFY YOUR EMOTIONAL NEEDS

1. Track your day like a ledger and make a table with two columns.
2. In the Deposit column, identify energy replenishers and make a list of things that you enjoy doing, those that energize you and/or relax you and recharge your battery. These might be solo or quiet time, hyperfocus activities or stimming (repetitive movements or sounds that help regulate emotions or sensory input).
3. Attach a value to the items on this list out of 100.
4. In the Withdrawal column, identify energy drainers and make a list of the things that stress you out, that you don't enjoy and that regularly drain you of energy. These might be loud environments, meetings, or sensory overload.
5. Attach a value to the items on this list out of 100.

Here's an example:

| DEPOSIT<br>= What recharges my battery (+) | WITHDRAWAL<br>= What uses up my energy (−) |
|---|---|
| Yoga (50)<br>Adequate nutrition (40)<br>Drinking adequate water (40)<br>Jacuzzi and sauna (30)<br>Soothing music (70)<br>Meditation (30)<br>Massage (30)<br>Adequate sleep (70)<br>Nature (50)<br>Creative activities (50)<br>My work (40)<br>Meeting a friend for coffee (30)<br>One-on-one time with my children (70)<br>Cuddles (90)<br>Sunshine (80) | Not sleeping well (70)<br>Crowds (60)<br>Loud noises (80)<br>Smelly things and places (90)<br>Bad music (90)<br>Heat (80)<br>Appointments (50)<br>Sensory overload from parenting two children on my own (90)<br>Socializing (50)<br>Screentime (40)<br>Rushing (40)<br>Lack of sunshine (80) |
| Total + | Total − |

6. Once a week, make a new table with these two columns and jot down the things you've done in the week that energize you (the Deposits) and those that drain you (the Withdrawals).
7. Add up the values in each column.
8. Use your final scores to help you spot patterns and understand when burnout is creeping in.
9. Decide if you need to do more things to add to the score in the Deposits column, for example planning recovery time if you know a high-energy cost event is coming up.
10. Balance out your day and week so your total energy doesn't fall too far into the negative. Being constantly in the red will lead to overwhelm or shutdown.

## COMPASSION-FOCUSED THERAPY

As you continue to process what has happened to you during the course of your late-diagnosis journey, you may have fresh insights into how your past continues to influence the way you show up in the present.

Here's the conundrum. So many of us have survived traumatic episodes by disconnecting from the emotions we felt when the wounding took place. We've numbed ourselves in order to survive. If past traumatic events instilled fear within us at the time, then reliving traumatic episodes from our past without a trained neurodivergent-affirming therapist can elicit a fear response in our present and re-traumatize us. As someone who underwent trauma therapy for over a year and a half, I can vouch for this and would agree that therapy can be incredibly tough on the mind and body.

If you are considering therapy, you need to ask yourself if it's something you are ready for and what you can do to balance all the heaviness that could potentially arise from processing your emotional history. Start by asking yourself:

- Are you ready for this? The emotional processing can add psychological stress on your nervous system, actually increasing any inflammation that needs to be eliminated.
- Do you have an adequate support system outside of therapy to ground you in your present reality?
- Can you handle this amid all of life's demands?
- If you've already started therapy, do you need to take a break from it?
- Is there an alternative therapy that doesn't involve talking about trauma, and you may prefer to widen your window of tolerance through other means?

If you are ready to dare to excavate beyond the layers of conditioning and address the emotional wounds that keep you from showing up as your authentic self, I would always suggest compassion-focused psychotherapy to help you gain self-awareness and self-compassion. Be sure to seek out a good therapist (see box below).

### How to Identify a Good Therapist

A good therapist has the following qualities:

- You have a good rapport and feel safe with them.
- They are compassionate.
- They are non-judgemental of the labels you identify with and use the information associated with the labels to support your emotional processing and recovery.
- They challenge you in the right way but don't try to influence your actions.
- They help you build healthy coping strategies to manage your challenges.
- They leave you in an emotionally regulated state at the end of the session.

## Tailored Therapy

As some neurodivergents have suffered from PTSD, therapy can be tailored to suit them through the following approaches:

**Compassionate inquiry:** a psychotherapeutic approach developed by Dr Gabor Maté, which looks beneath the surface of our behaviours to find the source of our struggles without any blame attached to the individual.

**Psychoeducation:** providing a clear outline of what to expect in therapy and tailoring this to the neurodivergent's accessibility needs, such as recording the sessions to enable playback, using video, audio or drawing to illustrate the points discussed in therapy.

**Engaging in special interests:** many neurodivergents, especially autistic individuals, have highly focused and absorbing interests, which can be a very welcome and effective self-soothing tool when attempting to recover from sensory meltdowns.

**Noticing what recounting trauma does to the body:** recalling difficult memories can elicit a trauma response that manifest as shortness of breath or pain in distinct parts of the body. Your therapist should be able to help you regulate your emotions and come back to ventral vagal (connection) state.

**Recognizing alexithymia or dyslexithymia:** both neurodivergence and trauma can create difficulties in describing experiences, and we may at times use the wrong words in doing this too. Therapists need to be able to ask the right questions to get to the answer they need.

**Differentiating sensory triggers from traumatic triggers:** neurodivergents may encounter sensory meltdowns rather than a traumatic trigger, so it's important to recognize the sensory root cause as traditional trauma coping methods won't work.

**Integration of the Self:** many neurodivergents who were traumatized tend to experience a fragmentation of the Self, where different parts within themselves are at war with one another. A neurodivergent-affirming therapist can help the individual recognize the parts within themselves. Rather than needing to banish these parts, it's about finding your most authentic manifestation and using this as a manual to guide you in different life situations going forward.

Therapy is difficult for anyone, let alone us neurodivergents who feel so intensely, so some sessions can be incredibly emotional as we uncover the sadness, shame, fear and guilt associated with our belief system.

In my journey to find emotional safety within myself, I've tried working on myself alone, with a therapist, in a community and with people I trust and who care deeply for me. I found that the most significant shifts happen not via the moment-to-moment emotional regulation techniques, but in achieving an integrative state via long-term psychotherapy, meditation and psychedelics-assisted therapy.

In this state, my ego dissolved and I began to see myself and my role in the relationships in my life. I was able to see my sense of self in its purest form, where the shell I'd developed to protect me fell apart. It felt like I'd always been there and I could finally breathe easy. Breaking free helped me see the world through child-like wonder.

However, please note that psychedelic-assisted therapy is not generally recommended for individuals with a personal or family history of schizophrenia, schizoaffective disorder, bipolar I disorder or other psychotic conditions. These substances can increase the risk of triggering psychosis or mania, particularly in genetically vulnerable individuals. Caution is also advised for those with unstable cardiovascular conditions, epilepsy or untreated severe trauma that may destabilize under intense emotional experiences.

### How to Protect Yourself in Therapy

1. Adopt self-regulation tools such as breathwork, yoga and Pilates. You can practise these trauma-release exercises in between your sessions to help widen your window of tolerance.
2. Prioritize energy recovery via a healthy sleep routine, adequate nutrition that helps rid the body of inflammation,

> stress reduction and exercise. Be mindful of sensory stimuli as recounting traumatic events can heighten our sensory sensitivity.
> 3. Self-soothe using positive coping strategies such as connecting with family and friends, being in nature, and other activities that give you healthy dopamine. It may be tempting to reach for old and unhealthy coping strategies!

## REDISCOVER THE POWER OF PLAY

In *The Myth of Normal*,[13] Gabor Maté describes four irreducible needs of children.

1. **An attachment relationship:** as we saw in Step 4, this entails forming a deep sense of contact and connection with our caregiver.
2. **Rest:** a sense of attachment and security that allows the child to be themselves and rest from having to work to make someone else happy.
3. **Validating of emotion:** permission to feel one's emotions, to have the safety to remain vulnerable, to be attended to for who we are not what we do.
4. **Play:** experience of free play to attain emotional, social and intellectual growth.

Here's the deal. As children, when we suppress authenticity in exchange for attachment, we adapt to do what is in the best interest of others. And it doesn't end in childhood. This mindset influences our behaviour, and when repeated over time, can become a deeply ingrained habit.

Then, one day, you wake up as somebody who gives so much to those around you, who is a 'nice' people-pleaser. You've never learned to ask for what you need, so you don't voice your needs until you feel angry and disappointed at being ignored. And when you do voice your authentic needs, it will be very likely met with dismissal and strong emotions from your partners and family. Or you may even develop hyper-expectations in your relationships, expecting them to fill the void left from your unmet attachment needs and incomplete emotional development.

This begins to create instability in your relationships and when conflict ensues, it makes you doubt yourself. You withdraw. You lash out. *Am I not enough? Am I too much?* Why would your partner accommodate your needs when there's a very good chance that they were in the relationship in the first place because they were looking to *YOU* to meet their needs? You internalize their disapproval as a personal character flaw and feel depleted of energy, because you just don't know how to express your emotions in a mature enough way that'll allow the both of you to resolve the conflict. When our emotions become stuck in our minds and body, we can feel lost and alone.

Healing your unhealthy emotional patterns begins to take shape the day you own who you are and what you want. And with this also comes the possibility of needing to leave some relationships behind as you become more authentic. So many of us have lived for others for so long that we have forgotten to live for ourselves.

You may find yourself beginning to exercise the release of stifled emotional energy within you and do more of what makes you feel alive. I know this chapter has been pretty serious, but I'd now like to end Step 5 by looking at some of the fun that we can bring into our lives – through the power of play.

The default mode of a child is to play. When we play, we come out of survival mode. Play is one of the most sophisticated social connections, as it requires us to participate in an activity and in most instances, to communicate our thoughts and intention. And through play, we can:

- Reclaim a sense of agency, control and feeling of safety.
- Express our pent-up emotions and heal.
- Reconnect with our bodies and integrate our senses.
- Build connection and feel part of a community.
- Foster resilience and empowerment.

## A Play Menu

For neurodivergents, a play menu can could include some of the following:

- Interests such as cooking, baking, learning about human behaviours, cinema.
- Creative expression such as writing, art, music, theatre, dance, photography.
- Altruism and focusing on a mission-driven purpose like creating a supportive community based on a shared goal, or working on a project that makes a difference to others.
- Spiritual practices such as yoga, meditation, mindfulness, breathwork, prayer.
- Nature, including forest bathing, walking, running, gardening.
- Endurance sports like long-distance running, marathon, triathlon, kayaking, skiing.
- Exercise and games such as swimming, strength training, cardio, horse riding, puzzles, board games, role-playing games.
- Spending time with pets.
- Travelling.

## Find Your Fun

What does fun look like to you? If you find yourself stuck for an answer, perhaps the following will help:

1. What makes you feel joy and alive?
2. If you don't see this in your current life, go back to your childhood and ask yourself, what did you enjoy? Did you have any interests and hobbies?

> 3. If you have a child, what activities do you expose them to that you enjoy too?
> 4. What does it take to weave fun and play into your daily life? What can you do to make it happen?

## What Play Looks Like for Me

For me, play means being in a flow state, expressing myself creatively, learning about new concepts relating to our neurodivergent way of being, spiritual practices, travelling to far-flung places, spending time with people who stimulate my mind and are good for my nervous system, and focusing on my purpose in life.

We know that emotions can take hold intensely in our mind and body and become stuck there. But when we are in a state of flow, our emotions can then morph into dynamic energies that flow like a river from inside us and out into the world.

Yoga has been one of the ways I've begun to play again. When I attend a class with others who turned up to the practice for their own reasons, I feel like a part of a community with a common purpose to resolve whatever we've faced that day. Each breath and every movement I take help me align the thoughts and feelings coursing through my veins and in my mind. By the end of the class, rather than feeling as though the different parts of myself are at war, I feel more at peace, as though the thoughts and emotions are flowing through me rather than to me.

I've also done a few solo trips abroad this year to awaken the free spirit that has lain dormant within me. And I took my kids on holiday to visit friends where we made some beautiful memories. Seeing them sat at the front of a speedboat as their hair blew in the wind and feeling a part of a community who genuinely care for one another made me feel awestruck. The journey from finding out I am an ADHDer, to realizing it was actually AuDHD I was dealing with, the unpacking of the trauma, the shedding of the heavy layer that I piggybacked into every corner of my life, and then travelling full circle home to myself has been nothing short of extraordinary.

In the last two or three years, I've plunged headfirst into play, into daring to do what I had feared, not always by choice and at times more out of necessity – and I've not regretted any of it. So many of us neurodivergents do things for the fascinating stories that we'll live to tell afterwards, even if it may not seem obvious to us at the time. Because what is more important to us than the need to feel alive? And as part of feeling alive, our relationships with ourselves and those around us have their own important roles to play.

# Step 6:
# Expect Your Relationships to Change and Adapt

By this point in our exploration of the layers of the ADHD iceberg, I hope you've begun to understand a little more about your physical and emotional needs as a neurodivergent. You may also become more aware of the external elements that can impact your internal states. Initially, you may find that this new self-awareness starts to go into overdrive whenever your neurodivergent traits come into focus. It could feel as though you have an X-ray vision into how your level of self-esteem has been driving your behaviour over all those years, including the choices you made, the partners you chose, and the quality of the relationships you've had, which in turn has helped to determine your levels of happiness. As author and psychotherapist Esther Perel says, 'The quality of your relationships determines the quality of your life.'[1]

It's only natural that when we begin to discover who we really are, our relationship with ourselves begins to change, too. We may also start to evaluate our other relationships in light of how we show up in the world. We become more aware of what our coping strategies are, and we may start to unmask in our closest relationships.

In Step 6, we're going to look at how our relationships can evolve once we start understanding ourselves as ADHDers and our real needs. As change and times of transition can be tricky for us to navigate, I'll be sharing some coping strategies with you too. And I will be focusing on four types of relationship that call for your most urgent attention in your neurodivergent journey.

1. Your relationship with yourself
2. Romantic relationships
3. Familial relationships
4. Social relationships

I'll be exploring the common relationship issues we face that we need to be mindful of, the most frequently asked questions around relationships in my community talks, and what relationships might mean for us.

## IN LOVE WITH LOVE

I have to confess that I've always put romantic relationships on a pedestal. Whenever things got turbulent for me while I was growing up, I would withdraw into romantic novels and inhale every word that painted a rich world of connection, tragedy, despair and love. To me, love still has a spiritual quality to it, a transcendent means of elevating us out of our deepest pains into connection.

Today, when it comes to romantic relationships, I feel like I've spent much of my life adrift at sea, looking for an anchor – for someone or something to ground that restless spirit within me. To make me feel complete, to make me feel like I mattered, because deep down, I didn't believe I did. I was genuinely surprised when boys liked me. As someone who was so starved of love, I sought validation in their admiration and felt truly seen for the first time.

It was not until I turned 18 that I had my first boyfriend, and I've not been single for long ever since, except for the one year when my best friend fulfilled the role usually taken up by a boyfriend. We'd gone to New York together and posed next to a colourful shop window with a neon tag that read 'Friends are forever, boys are whatever'. However, that friendship sadly wasn't forever either.

Within a relationship, I took on the shape of whomever I was with – without a steady sense of who I really was. I became all-giving in what was needed to maintain that connection and projected my ideal partner onto whomever I was dating. Then just as quickly as the rush of love came, it would subside without any warning. I would wake up one day feeling like a barrel that had been drained of all its contents. I was and still am highly sensitive to the emotions, thoughts and moods of those around me, and the vibes of places I find myself in. Perhaps it is because of this that I felt that I needed someone to shield me from the world.

This need intensified when I moved halfway around the world to set up on my own. Even though I had some great, stable partners, I also seemed to have a knack for attracting dark and wounded souls that saw me as a refuge for their pain. Without a steady sense of self, I adapted to what the other person in each of those relationships wanted. It was unthinkable for me to say no, and I also didn't know how to ask for what I needed. I would get upset, anxious or depressed when I felt that my needs weren't being fulfilled.

Later in life, once diagnosed with ADHD and ASD, I came to see how common it is for neurodivergents to struggle in relationships – whether professionally, romantically or socially. Why do we often show up in our relationships like children, even when our livelihood depends on our maturity in our workplaces and our homes?

Through being embroiled in my own relationship dramas and those of my friends, I saw that even the most kind, righteous, intelligent and beautiful people you will ever meet in your life can be emotionally immature. And that includes myself. This is why I think 'intention' can be such a loaded word, because even if we set out with the intention to do our best in a relationship, it seems that when we're faced with triggers that set off our autonomic stress response, we are powerless... unless we find such radical self-acceptance that we're able to break free from the chains of our emotional history, knowing that the only person we have always needed to love us, is us.

## HEALING IN OUR RELATIONSHIPS WITH OTHERS

As a community, we have our work cut out for us on our emotional journey – not least because we're sensitive to the world due to our unique biological states, which can change from moment to moment. On top of this, some of us may fluctuate emotionally and mentally between shame and grandiosity in different relational contexts. And if that weren't enough, we find ourselves living at a time in Western history that is steeped in a patriarchal, individualistic and anti-relational culture.

However, many of us are slowly finding our way back to ourselves, learning to recognize relationships and environments that no longer support our wellbeing. While not everyone has the means or security to enable them to leave difficult situations, more and more of us are beginning to question patterns of self-betrayal and tune inward to listen to our own needs. This shift invites a new kind of honesty – one that values what feels right for 'me', even if that sometimes sits in tension with what's expected of 'us'.

But how do we heal alone, when we need each other? As Terry Real, founder of Relational Life Foundation, which teaches a revolutionary approach to couples therapy, says, 'Nothing is more important in our lives than our relationships. A great relationship boosts your immune system, opens your heart, and keeps you vital and creative.'[2]

Often, trauma stems from a violation in a relationship, an emotional rupture when we've had to deal with what is happening within us by disconnecting from ourselves to survive, or disconnecting from others to protect ourselves.

I think this is why our most intimate relationships can bring up our unhealed wounds. And to heal, we need to correct our experience in relational repair. Trauma heals in connection, but is it that easy? No.

I don't know if anyone can claim that they've cracked it in relationships. The nature of relationships is that they involve connecting with another person, and if you think about how hard it is to understand what you need, it's even harder to figure out what another person needs so all parties continue to feel validated and connected. We're all learning and adapting. Relationship is a skill, not a given, and for any relationship to work, there are some basic yet crucial skills we need to master.

- Listening
- Finding a shared vision
- Communicating your needs in a caring way
- Commitment to showing up better and making it work
- Negotiation

Sounds simple, doesn't it? If only it was...

## MOST COMMON ISSUES IN NEURODIVERSE RELATIONSHIPS

Make no mistake, in any relationship, the layers that underlie the surface of every interaction are profound. As Terry Real remarks in his trainings on Relational Life Therapy, there is the adult self, but also the wounded child and adaptive child at play in our significant relationships.

We've all had challenging things happen to us, and some of us might have had the tools to deal with them. For those of us who didn't and who are born with neurological differences, there can be a gap in understanding the people we have relationships with, whether romantic or otherwise, due to our communication differences. And even if we do understand them, but they refuse to work with us due to their own issues around opening up to another person, then it's a no-go too.

Here's just a few examples of how we differ in the way we process information as neurodivergents:

- How we perceive others' actions
- How fast we process information
- How we react instinctively before we can reflect
- How we deal with others when we don't fully understand them
- How we take feedback on board
- How we recover from being misunderstood

Because of this, when we face triggers, our reactions in the moment may not be the best representation of our adult self. In addition to this, our differences as neurodivergents can lead to misunderstanding and misinterpretations (see box below).

Once we have an understanding of these potential issues, we can be more aware of them arising in our own relationships. This doesn't mean we should be ashamed if they do, as that could just trap us even more deeply in a cycle of low-esteem. It just means that if we happen to notice them, we can think about how we are going to address them and then take the appropriate action, such as talking to the other person, or finding the professional support we need to help us navigate our relationships in healthy ways.

The realization that, unbeknownst to us, our neurodivergent differences have been playing out in our relationships can be a lot to take on board. And if you've recently received an ADHD diagnosis, you may also find yourself re-examining your relationships in light of this, too – not least of all your relationship with yourself.

---

### Common Difficulties with Relationships

**Executive function differences:** daily struggles in maintaining living space, getting out on time, planning and organizing.

**Difficulty understanding people's intentions (theory of mind deficit):** leads to misunderstanding of non-verbal cues, and therefore difficulty reciprocating a social connection.

**Emotional dysregulation:** difficulty processing emotions and possibility of emotional outbursts or avoiding conflict.

**Rejection sensitivity dysphoria:** feeling rejected at feedback, even when it's meant to be healthy.

**Alexithymia:** having no words for a feeling, and inaccurate communication of our emotions and thoughts.

**Affective empathy:** being susceptible to absorbing the emotions of others, adding overwhelm to our senses.

> - **Impulsivity:** impulsive actions can lead to misunderstanding or the other person feeling that their needs are neglected.
> - **Sensory overwhelm:** often heightened when we process emotions via therapy, as the emotional circuits are also closely linked to sensory circuits in the brain.
> - **Hyper-fixation on special interests:** our partners may feel neglected when we over-focus on our interest or info-dump something they have no interest in, leading to one-sided conversations.
> - **Low frustration tolerance:** lower levels of patience and being quick to anger.
> - **Limerence or person addiction:** an intense and involuntary obsession, infatuation and desire for a person that can lead us to neglect the rest of our lives.
> - **Unhealthy attachment styles:** insecure, anxious, avoidant, fearful or disorganized attachment style formed from childhood or our current relationships which can get in the way of forming healthy relationships.
> - **Hyper-sexuality, asexuality or hypo-sexuality:** a mismatch in sexual compatibility can create a disconnect or resentment in romantic relationships over time.

## UNPACKING YOUR NEURODIVERGENT LABEL WHILE IN A RELATIONSHIP

Imagine waking up one day, realizing that you've been a mystery wrapped in an enigma to yourself. You seem to have focused outwards all your life, ensuring that everyone else around you is okay without stopping to think about what you need.

Deep down, you know you matter, but you've likely messed up more than once and you are scared to face what you know you have to face. You may not trust yourself to know what you need, or have the courage and skills to ask for it. And then the conflicts happen, and you aren't proud of the way you act in response. You don't understand why it's so hard for you to just say what you mean, and you end up saying what you don't mean instead.

The first 12 to 24 months after diagnosis can be one of the most challenging times in a neurodivergent's life. It's apparently one of life's significant traumas to get a health diagnosis late in life, and they say you can go through a grief cycle when you come to terms with a diagnosis such as ADHD in adulthood. I can imagine why: you're very likely suddenly exposed to an onslaught of information on the internet about who you supposedly are, while not having the tools to fully understand how to make sense of this information and make yourself feel better.

When you combine this with starting therapy or medication while not knowing how these will affect how you show up, you could find yourself simultaneously dismantling old patterns while trying to rebuild. Some call this chaos, while others deem it to be a transitional rite of passage to self-transformation. Which camp will you find yourself in? Whether you are a glass half full or glass half empty person, it's a life shake-up that will affect not only you, but everyone in your vicinity. You're changing, and it's best you know what you're in for.

You will most probably embark on a journey that starts with recalling every major or minor event in which you were confused about the way you acted, while trying to understand who you are, what you need, and renegotiating these needs with those closest to you. If the foundations of your relationships are strong enough, there's every chance you can weather this storm together. However, if your relationships are built on fragile foundations, such as inauthenticity, there's a chance you may start to feel like the life you've created for yourself is far removed from what you need for the wellbeing of your authentic self.

Similar to the grief cycle, these are the stages you could go through:

## 1. Denial

- Not accepting of the information within the label – and why should you, when parts of it don't seem to relate to you?
- Insistence on the superpower narrative for neurodivergence.
- You may reject the medical model and pour your denial back into the world through living a life of purpose, doubling down on advocacy in your sphere of influence, and offering support to others before you take any care of yourself.

## 2. Anger/Fear

- Anger at yourself for masking and anger at your parents, too, for not recognizing what was going on (it may not all be their fault, but this is how anger works – it can spring from a lack of personal freedom).
- Anger at current partner or even your children for not making the effort to understand or support you better.
- Sometimes, this stage can elicit a stress response that makes certain people combative and refuse to take personal responsibility for how this can make others feel.
- Not accessing support for fear of being stigmatized.
- Anger at others who don't seem to understand.

## 3. Bargaining

- Wanting to understand what your authentic needs are and where your coping strategies began.
- Unmasking with no apologies made, temporarily forgetting we still need connection with others to be happy, and therefore still need to make some compromises in our relationships.
- Attempting to over-explain the reasons behind your behaviour in a bid to seek understanding, or not at all.
- Debating the possible outcomes of asking for adjustments – whether you will be understood or be infantilized.

### 4. Depression

- Experiencing physical, mental and emotional burnout from advocating for yourself or others.
- Feeling isolated if others do not seem to understand or accept you.
- Feeling disconnected, lost and despairing, preferring to spend time alone.
- Desire to find like-minded people who understand and accept you.

### 5. Acceptance

- Understanding your needs and advocating for yourself.
- Recognizing your strengths.
- Being compassionate and kind when the parts of you that are hard to love arise.
- Knowing how to tap into tools to support your regulation.
- Making sense of your past.
- Working on your triggers and finding closure with the traumatic events that happened to you.
- Upgrading your relationship with yourself, based on authenticity and acceptance.
- Feeling loved and a deep sense of belonging when validated for your struggles, seen as human and accepted.
- Learning to connect with others while asserting your social and emotional needs.

It's not a given that you will experience all or indeed any of these emotions in this order, or that they won't return in another guise later. Grief looks different for different people, and there is no wrong or right way to feel, as feelings can come and go. It's all part of the ongoing journey towards self-awareness and self-acceptance following a diagnosis.

### Reflection

If you have recently received an ADHD diagnosis, could the grief cycle help you to explain what you are experiencing to your loved ones?

## HOW STARTING MEDICATION CAN AFFECT RELATIONSHIPS

I'd like to take a brief look at what starting medication can do while coming to terms with a diagnosis of ADHD later in life.

As described in Step 3, for some, medication is life-changing. When it works, it's like putting on a pair of glasses that focus everything in view, where previously the picture was hazy. Things feel a little brighter, more surmountable, and you may feel calmer and, dare I say, happier.

But while it works well for many, for those with a more complex neurobiological landscape, such as the AuDHD experience, the medication may upset the neurotransmitter balance and impact how they show up mentally, emotionally and socially. For example, for an AuDHDer with variable levels of dopamine and norepinephrine in the prefrontal area of the brain, starting a stimulant medication that increases these neurotransmitter levels might mean that you may at times have higher neurotransmitter levels than you need. It can enhance your monotropism – your capacity for tunnel vision – and you may find it difficult to break that hyper-focus, while getting annoyed with those around you who try to pull you away from whatever is holding your interest. In this state, you're all about getting absorbed in a flow state, and less about the relationships around you.

A few other considerations also come to mind:

- If you have higher levels of dopamine, being on a dose that may be too high for you some of the time, combined with your overstimulated dopamine receptors, may eventually lead to increased tolerance to medication. You may find yourself being less motivated or having low frustration tolerance, and incorrectly thinking you need to increase your medication dosage.
- For those with reduced catecholamine metabolism, for example AuDHDers, increasing norepinephrine may increase sympathetic activation over a prolonged period. This may cause you to act like

you're running from danger, increasing your drive to achieve, and may make you appear more intense to those around you.

- For many neurodivergent women – particularly those undergoing major hormonal transitions such as puberty, pregnancy, perimenopause or hormone replacement therapy (HRT) – elevated oestrogen levels can increase dopamine activity in the brain. When stimulant medications are introduced during these periods, dopamine levels may rise too high, leading to overstimulation. This can manifest as intense hyperfocus and increased sympathetic nervous system activity (i.e., the fight-or-flight response), raising the risk of burnout. Because your hormonal landscape shifts week to week, there may be times when oestrogen levels exceed your body's optimal threshold. This can result in oestrogen dominance, where the body struggles to metabolise and eliminate excess oestrogen. Symptoms of this imbalance may include mood swings, weight gain, bloating, headaches, fatigue and heightened distractibility or hyperactivity.

The above are just a few examples of the realities of many neurodivergents who start medication later in life, and who may feel better to begin with, but then gradually sense that the helpful effects are starting to wear off. While your body is adjusting to the new medications, this will also have an effect on your mind and how you show up from moment to moment in your relationships. I've lost count of the number of ADHDers who've told me that when their focus is enhanced, they can find it hard to balance their attention between work and romantic partners, family responsibilities and even fun, causing conflicts in their relationships.

In addition, if you start therapy on top of taking medication, you may find yourself being more sensitive to sensory triggers in your daily life, because our sensory inputs are linked to emotional responses. This is okay if you work for yourself and are generally in control of your environment. But as some of us still need to go into the office some of the time, we may unwittingly end up experiencing sensory overwhelm, which might look like an exaggerated emotional response to those around us.

If we are aware of how our physical, mental and emotional states may change, we will gain more self-awareness and self-compassion, but we may also need more compassion from others. If you aren't sure how your authentic self will be received by others, the interactions at this time can be fraught with uncertainties.

When we think about how we all bring our own unique triggers and need for safety into our relationships, perhaps it's not surprising that our relationships will change and we will need to adapt. And sometimes, the way we show up may confuse those in relationships with us.

Of course, relationships themselves are confusing enough to navigate without the added factor of ADHD, as we can't always be sure of what other issues we might be dealing with that originate with the other person. It's also important to understand that we're not always to blame. We may often enter into relationships with another neurodivergent, but perhaps we're the one whose condition was identified first and we may therefore carry the burden of the label.

## ADHD AND THE RISE OF PERSONALITY DISORDERS

When I give talks to neurodivergent audiences, there is a question that comes up again and again: 'How do I avoid attracting a narcissist?' Just to be clear, the people who ask this question include men, women, non-binary individuals and other gender identities. And the context isn't just in romantic relationships. I've heard about neurodivergents referring to their parents or even managers as narcissists too. Given that this label is perhaps used a little too freely for anyone who seems to behave in ways we can't understand, we also have to ask why we might feel so victimized by the actions of another.

While many neurodivergents are indeed vulnerable to unhealthy relationships, and it is often much better for our health and wellbeing to be out of them, we must also learn to recognize what we're dealing with exactly. Is it a narcissistic personality disorder (NPD) or a borderline personality disorder (BPD) with irredeemable qualities – or are we perhaps dealing with someone else with a divergent mind who is still using the adaptive traits that they learned from their childhood, which are now becoming maladaptive in their adult relationships? Or perhaps we're being a little too quick to point a finger at others? Now, my intention here is not to excuse behaviours, but to provide explanations. However, I draw the line at using our neurodivergence as an excuse to cause harm to others – that's not okay.

In recent years, many neurodiversity advocates have questioned whether what we sometimes think of as NPDs or any other personality disorders (PDs) are in fact individuals with autism or ADHD who have an underlying history of trauma or neglect, and who show up with anger issues or conflict-avoidant tendencies when their stress response is triggered. These terms can often be misused and sensationalized, when the reality of the presentation can be nuanced.

A recent study broadly concluded that ADHDers are ten times more likely to be narcissists themselves, and that women with ADHD are more frequently diagnosed with BPD and histrionic personality disorder.[3] The study acknowledged that these findings may not be accurate, as the shared symptoms between BPD and the torturous self-regard of narcissistic vulnerability may have skewed the results. The authors warned the public not to draw any concrete conclusions from their findings, which they admitted to be highly generalized in relation to the ADHD community as a whole.

Nevertheless, perhaps we need to rethink our approach to labels like NPD? In Terry Real's Relational Life Therapy, he simplifies the labels down to how someone is presenting in unsavoury ways in a relationship. So instead of the label 'narcissist', he looks at the layer underneath this – which is grandiosity and shame.

On the surface, someone who's deemed a narcissist often shows the following behaviours:

- Lacking empathy
- Inflated sense of self-importance

# STEP 6: EXPECT YOUR RELATIONSHIPS TO CHANGE AND ADAPT

- Sense of entitlement and being preoccupied with fantasies around success, beauty and status
- Grandiosity
- Low self-esteem
- Manipulating others to achieve an aim
- Need for admiration
- Sensitive to criticisms or perceived rejection

Underneath this persona, grandiosity impairs judgement, blunts empathy and distorts a realistic assessment of negative consequences.

Narcissism is perhaps the most misunderstood personality trait in some respects, as it can often arise from the need for control that is born out of inflexibility and fear. In fact, these are some of the lesser-known traits associated with narcissism:

- People-pleasing
- Self-serving behaviours, such as prioritizing their own wellbeing at the expense of others (yes, it is important to love ourselves, but not at the expense of mistreating or hurting others)
- Can be empathetic and well-meaning but so concerned with how other people perceive them that they become obsessively self-centred and anxious – hello, people-pleasers!

## Who are Narcissists Attracted to?

Everyone and anyone who's had a relationship with a narcissist will tell you that they are attracted to empaths.

An empath is often a highly sensitive person who is capable of deep emotional understanding, starved of love and tends to fall in love deeply and quickly. As an empath, you could be self-confident when you're on your own, but when you fall in love, you take on your partner's energy to the degree where your sense of self is determined by how they see you, how well they care for you, and how happy they are.

So do I personally believe in these labels? The more I heal and remove myself from a sense of victimhood in my own relationships, the more I see that this pairing can attract each other in order to heal the wounds that may become re-exposed through unhealthy relationship dynamics. For example, I once dated someone who held onto me for fear of doing life alone, even when he didn't have the energy or desire to commit to our relationship. Did I blame him for this blatant selfishness? No, because I had a similar fear. The difference was, I believe in being fair and living my life as honestly as possible. It can be incredibly heart-breaking when you realize that not everyone adheres to the same value system, but we have to learn to tackle these situations with self-awareness and to understand our own part in perpetuating unhealthy relationships.

## CONNECTIONS BETWEEN ADHD PERSONALITY TRAITS AND PERSONALITY DISORDERS

According to the Royal College of Psychiatrists, a personality disorder is defined as 'an enduring condition which interferes with the sufferer's sense of wellbeing and ability to function in full in ordinary social settings.'[24] Keeping this definition in mind, when might the way we act and our ADHD personality traits cross over to become a personality disorder?

In trait theory, which is one approach to personality in psychology, the Big Five traits that make up personality include the following groupings:

1. **Extroversion:** sociability and assertiveness
2. **Openness to experience:** creative imagination
3. **Emotional stability (neuroticism):** anxiety
4. **Agreeableness:** compassion and respect
5. **Conscientiousness:** responsibility and organization

These traits exist on a spectrum, and many autistic individuals and ADHDers have personality traits that could seem like personality disorders to the untrained eye. In fact, many members of our community have been given personality disorder labels, such as borderline personality disorder (BPD), either informally by those who live with us or formally by clinicians. However, most people don't fit neatly into one label, as our traits can ebb and flow, and I would hazard a guess that the archetypal person with BPD, as defined by psychiatry, probably doesn't look much like you or I on any given day.

All the same, how do we tell the difference between neurodivergence and a personality disorder? Many of the traits of personality disorders and ASD overlap; for example, a person with a personality disorder may have an unstable and incoherent sense of identity, a 'chameleon-like' identity, that is similar to the traits that somebody with ASD can form as a result of masking in order to function in different settings. Personally, I feel the definition of personality disorder is deeply flawed, as it doesn't reflect the richness and complexity of what it means to be human. I see myself in that 'chameleon' description: someone with a shapeshifter persona, constantly adapting to different spaces. But to me, that's not a disorder – it's just who I am and coming to terms with.

The DSM-5 (*Diagnostic and Statistical Manual of Mental Disorders*) states that personality disorders typically develop in adolescence to early adulthood, while ADHD and autism start in early childhood. So, could living with undiagnosed ADHD and autism while adapting to emotional turmoil be a recipe for developing a personality disorder? Collecting a developmental history of the early presence or absence of ADHD or autistic features is vital for a conclusive diagnosis, including features that are typically camouflaged in women.

Research has shown that those who are diagnosed with personality disorders tend to fulfil the criteria to be diagnosed with ASD. Another study showed that 68 per cent of autistic individuals fulfil the diagnostic criteria of at least one personality disorder.[5] It seems that ADHDers also have a high incidence of personality disorders of over 52.4 per cent[6] (see box below).

## Common Personality Disorders in ADHDers and Autistic Individuals

**Dependent:** individuals feel they have an excessive need to be taken care of, leading to clinginess, fear of abandonment and difficulty making decisions independently.

**Depressive:** exhibit a range of depressive behaviours, such as chronic and enduring patterns of sadness, hopelessness and low self-esteem.

**Avoidant:** symptoms include excessive social anxiety and fear of intimacy and rejection.

**Borderline:** characterized by significant interpersonal relationship instability, a distorted sense of self, mood swings, fear of abandonment and intense emotional responses.

**Histrionic:** excessive attention-seeking, needing approval, dramatic, impulsive and extremely emotional.

**Negativistic:** passive-aggressive behaviours, including covert obstructionism.

**Antisocial:** manipulative, exploitative and showing lack of remorse.[7]

I've shared this list with you for information purposes only, as while these personality disorders have been documented among neurodivergent individuals, we're also learning that personality traits can change, so it's potentially not something that you are stuck with or even need to worry about! However, if anything in the list does ring any bells for you, remember that you don't have to struggle with any condition on your own, so do seek professional help.

## CAUSES OF MENTAL HEALTH CONDITIONS

Dr Chris Palmer, the Harvard psychiatrist and author of the acclaimed book *Brain Energy*, has explained that it's very hard to determine the root cause of mental health conditions, but in order for the brain to malfunction, the cells that regulate a host of neurological functions need to be either underactive, overactive or not functioning at all for a prolonged period of time.[8] As is the case in autism and ADHD, because they are neurodevelopmental conditions, if the neurons that control a certain brain function weren't developed, that function or signalling pathway will not exist. This is certainly true in the realms of social communication and interaction in both autistic individuals and personality disorders, which involve difficulties in forming and maintaining relationships, communicating our needs, and understanding both the self and others.[9] We can add to this the adaptations and neural pathways that become established from masking for many years, which in and of itself messes with our emotional regulation, sense of self and stress response.

When I took a deep dive into the clinical literatures comparing and contrasting ADHD, ASD and personality disorders, I couldn't help but think about how *permanent* personality disorders are often deemed to be in psychiatric research. While psychologists used to believe that personality traits are inherited and fixed, new research shows that they aren't – that it is possible for us to transform and intentionally embody new personalities well into adulthood.[10]

Dr Dan Siegel, a bestselling author and clinical professor of psychiatry at UCLA, surmises that personality development begins with our innate temperament, the neural tendencies that we are all born with, and is further influenced by our adaptations to the quality of our early attachment and our continuous life experiences. Dr Siegel has presented a new science-based, developmental and neurobiological framework for understanding personality called Patterns of Developmental Pathways (PDP).[11] Patterns of Developmental

Pathways takes a holistic approach which reveals the inner motivations driving the personality patterns we see on the surface.

PDP links three primal emotional systems, as described in neuroscientist Jaak Panksepp's work – anger, separation distress, and fear – with an infant's needs in the three domains of agency, bonding and certainty. When the drive for agency, bonding and certainty is frustrated, a baby's respective primary emotions of anger, separation distress and fear become activated. As personality disorders are usually described in a negative light, PDP is a more inclusive model which helps us investigate what happens when any of the three universal psychological needs becomes activated with a perceived lack:

1. **Agency for embodied empowerment:** empowers and uses the body and sense of existence to keep alive and well, bringing harmony, comfort and respect to self.
2. **Bonding for relational connection:** maintains a sense of connection that brings a sense of recognition, belonging, being seen, affection and receiving support.
3. **Certainty for prediction and safety:** attempts to detect danger and construct patterns to create safety and be prepared.

Personality patterns that appear conflicting are often the result of a lack of linkage between what we feel inwardly and how we express this on the outside.

Some people may also develop a more dominant pattern of behaviour, such as repeatedly showing up in the same way when faced with conflict or demands. For example, autistic individuals are often known to have a deep need for control or certainty. Early in life, an autistic infant is born with sensory integration differences whereby they are tasked with the job of integrating the senses perceived outside the body, while trying to make sense of the senses perceived inside the body. The sensory processing system is linked to the emotional system, so any positive sensory inputs increase positive emotions and vice versa. Herein lies an integration challenge, where a young autistic child is dealing simultaneously with a lot of chaos and inflexibility at the sensory level.

So even when autistic children learn that social connection is the most stimulating thing ever for a human being, they may avoid it due to the sensory challenges and rejection sensitivity in order to keep themselves in some kind of equilibrium, even if this goes against human nature itself. Their day-to-day existence then becomes about striving to achieve some kind of internal balance, and they aren't necessarily training their mirror neurons – brain cells that are thought to play a key role in empathy and social understanding by mirroring the actions and emotions of others – to pick up on other people's non-verbal cues, which are needed to form and maintain relationships.

But this isn't to say that every autistic identity is non-agile or that autistic individuals will develop a personality that is avoidant to social connection. Girls, women and other intersectional identities – especially in the presence of co-occurring conditions like AuDHD – have to learn to observe people, to give them what is needed in every interaction, and to mask. In fact, many autistic women are wired to be even more socially driven than neurotypical women, alongside the expectations placed on the female gender to be more socially inclined than the male. However, it could also be that they learn to be sociable in their own unique way and eventually learn to choose friends they can tolerate or share interests with.

It's interesting to see how more dominant personality types develop when our early experiences don't always fit well with what the world demands from us. For example, an AuDHDer with a deep need for control and certainty, together with the need for adventure and novel experiences, may find it hard to resolve the internal tug of war, which will have an impact on their relationships.

When behaviours are repeated over time, the neural pathways become strengthened and set in as a recurring pattern. Achieving wholeness via therapy isn't about suppressing certain patterns of behaviour, but about enabling our energy to enter a more harmonious and integrative state of flow in a system that promotes linkages between agency (the need to be autonomous), bonding (the need to connect), and certainty (knowing what lies ahead). The growth work here involves focusing on a different emotional pathway than the one we usually go down, and to do this often enough to ensure this pathway gets strengthened over time, leading to a different and more desirable outcome. From another perspective, if our inherent need is for autonomy, perhaps the growth lies in radical acceptance, being honest about who we are and what we want, and finding stability through embracing change and uncertainty?

Our ability to potentially reroute our emotional pathways makes me question how useful personality disorder labels actually are. Interestingly, in recent years, the psychiatrists Roger Mulder and Peter Tyrer have made a well-informed case for rejecting the scientific validity of a diagnosis such as borderline personality disorder (BPD) and they highlight instead the confusion and harm it causes the individuals who are given the label.[12] They suggest that a diagnosis of BPD, commonly associated with neurodivergent women, reflects more on the clinician's affective emotional state than a careful assessment. Their report describes the 'myriad negative interactions in human relationships that have caused far beyond personality function, extending from simple disagreement to total functional breakdown'.[13] According to their findings, with which I'm inclined to agree, the label doesn't help treatment but invites stigma.

Sometimes, I feel like I'm pushing a huge boulder up a hill by questioning the validity of the labels given to us and working to destigmatize them. There are so many negative preconceived notions about each of the labels, especially when personality disorders are included; for example, the very description 'borderline' is itself enough to traumatize anyone who receives it, and anyone with such a diagnosis would require so much strength and self-assurance from their partner to accept it, work with them and not to use it *against* them.

When neurodivergents are diagnosed with personality disorders, this stays with them, even if the symptoms can often wax and wane based on the qualities of their interactions, relationships and their biology. However, as the world adopts new modes of healing our traumas via psychedelic-assisted therapy and meditation – which can help facilitate new neural connections, deactivate the default mode network, change the epigenetic expression of genes that are involved in the stress response and integration within our brain and body systems – who's to say personality disorders or mental health disorders aren't fixable?[14]

If one of the core triggers for borderline personality disorder (BPD) – widely considered one of the most painful personality disorders – is a deep sensitivity to abandonment or rejection, then it makes sense that falling in love can feel especially vulnerable. In those moments, we can lose our sense of separateness, becoming emotionally enmeshed with the other person. Without clear boundaries, our sense of self can become blurred, and suddenly our worth feels tied to their affection or approval. We're no longer standing on solid ground – we're ebbing and flowing based on how they perceive us or make us feel. Instead of focusing on the labels, we should instead focus on our needs to feel safe, secure, autonomous and connected. To do this, we need to know how these wounds were sustained in the first place, and rewrite the narratives in our minds.

As the common denominator of all personality disorders is emotional dysregulation, we need to look at the source of ruptures in relationships that weren't repaired and how that left us feeling distressed, afraid, alone or invalidated, and how we may have then carried this into the next relationship.

Perhaps big life-changing events or trauma underlie an insecure attachment in the past, which affects our sense of self and how we perceive the behaviours of others today? Perhaps underneath those destructive behaviours that arise in the name of personality disorders lie insecure attachments that can be explained via our attachment styles and the neurochemistry that underlies this?

As to whether your relationship partner actually does have a personality disorder, I think our actions when we are backed into a corner speak volumes about our personal sense of integrity or cruelty – behaviours which have less to do with neurodivergence and more to do with one's inner temperament and adaptive strategies from our life experiences – the good, the bad and everything in between.

The fact is that while we may believe we've put childhood long behind us, many of us remain still stuck in the unhealthy attachment styles we learned as infants.

## BEHAVING LIKE ADULTS

Within every relationship, there is an opportunity for transformation, but we can only grow if we're able to see the role we're playing ourselves and put a stop to unhealthy patterns. The work that we need to do begins with upgrading our core beliefs about ourselves and our relationships.

Both the empath and the narcissist have similar wounds rooted in shame and the belief that they are unlovable. If you fall into the empath camp, maybe you were a parentified child (that is, a child who was forced to take on adult responsibilities, including looking after others emotionally) and you needed to scan your environment constantly to figure out what you had to do to feel safe? When things happened to you, the adults in your life didn't do what they ought to have done to help you, so you did your best to deal with the situation and perhaps even tried to solve their problems for them. The sense of abandonment you felt left a lasting wound from the shame of believing you weren't worthy enough to be loved. You grew up hoping you could change others, so that you could turn your partner into the adult who was never there for you. But it doesn't work like that. The coping mechanisms that you developed as a child aren't appropriate for who you are now. As an adult yourself, you may still be showing up like a child in your relationships.

Many of us never learn to grow up. If we haven't yet learned to create healthy boundaries, soon we find our lines are crossed and resentment builds, leading to a push-pull pattern when we encounter conflict in relationships. This can manifest as the loop of doom, where one partner appears as anxious in their attachment style and the other is a love avoidant, at any given time. It becomes incredibly dizzying when both partners simultaneously exhibit both attachment styles, otherwise known as the disorganized attachment style – an insecure attachment style that as many as one-third of ADHDers and many autistic individuals are likely to have.[15],[16] According to a 2023 study by the Attachment Project, disorganized attachment can look like erratic behaviours in response to stress or fear.

We may be adults, but when we encounter emotional triggers of rejection (criticism), distance (avoidance) or abandonment (such as not hearing from our partners who appear uninterested), we are going to find our stress response being activated, and we begin to act like children. Cue emotional dysregulation and the inability to make sense of what is happening. For so many adults with this insecure attachment style, you may be able to manage your work or friendship circle because you're able to control how much access people have to you, but there's nothing like an intimate relationship to conjure up your deep-seated fear of being hurt. It is more than likely, also, that our attachment patterns change in different relationships. To get a clearer picture, let's dig a little deeper into the different types of attachment style.

## ATTACHMENT STYLES OR NEURODIVERGENT TRAITS?

Studies indicate that genetics can account for up to 45 per cent of the variability in anxious attachment and 39 per cent in avoidant attachment styles, with the quality of early relationships, particularly with primary caregivers, considered the most significant factor in determining attachment style.[17] Environmental influences, such as parenting, trauma and early relational experiences, play a much larger role in shaping how a person develops their attachment style.

As we've seen, attachment styles arise from the way we developed an emotional bond with our caregivers in childhood. They can be broadly divided into two styles: secure attachment and insecure attachment.

A securely attached child has a healthier foundation from which to perceive themselves and others, while an insecurely attached child may have a more dismal view of themselves and others. This can cause them difficulties in starting and maintaining close relationships.

It's worth saying that not all parent misattunement is intentional, as even with the best of intentions, the ways in which our culture believes we should raise our children can lead to parents not meeting their children's needs. But it's not all nurture's problem either, as genetically, there could be challenges for both the parent and child who are both neurodivergents as touched upon in Step 4. Neurologically, the differences in our brain structures and function can impact our emotional regulation and behaviours in our interpersonal interactions. If a parent is prone to depression, anxiety, obsessive-compulsive behaviours or sensory challenges, they may find it difficult to validate and be present to meet their child's needs.

However, it's important to note that this isn't always the case, as the quality of a neurodiverse relationship relies on so many factors, such as social communication, emotional regulation and our sensory processing abilities, as well as the resources and support available to the parent. Some neurodivergent children are able to form secure attachments with their parents, and it helps that more of us are getting diagnosed later in life. What we learn about ourselves now can help us provide a more compassionate and fair space in which to raise our own kids if they are neurodivergent and face similar challenges, instead of raising them to neurotypical standards.

By the time we reach adulthood, our attachment styles may exist on a spectrum, much like our neurodiverse traits do. While it's commonly thought that our emotional needs are linked to our attachment styles, if you are a therapist working with neurodivergent adults, you will need to understand where neurodivergent traits cross over with sensory needs, and attachment styles begin. For example, autistics and ADHDers may become overwhelmed by sensory triggers and leave a social setting that they are expected to attend, with the result that they may then become misunderstood as being avoidant. In actual fact, they were simply overwhelmed and unable to communicate it to others in that moment.

The table below shows examples of insecure attachment styles and where we may find them in the neurodiverse community in general.[18,19]

| INSECURE ATTACHMENT STYLES AND TRAITS IN RELATIONSHIPS | COMMON IN | NEURODIVERSE TRAITS THAT MAY APPEAR AS THESE ATTACHMENT STYLES AND COMPOUND CHALLENGES IN RELATIONSHIPS |
|---|---|---|
| **Avoidant/dismissive** Developed from being consistently neglected and not having their needs met – where caregiver ignores or doesn't know what they need and gives the wrong thing. <br>• As children, they tend to play by themselves <br>• Hyper-independent <br>• Avoid getting close emotionally <br>• Tendency to dissociate <br>• Being overly focused on one's own needs and comforts <br>• Withdrawal from unpleasant conversations or conflict | ADHD (inattentive presentation); autistic individuals | • Challenges with reading verbal or non-verbal cues lead to appearing blasé and emotionless <br>• Rigidity in sticking to routines and interests leads to lack of flexibility <br>• Social anxiety may lead to wanting to keep to ourselves <br>• Alexithymia or having no word to describe the way you're feeling can make you seem elusive to others <br>• Delayed mental processing leads to delay in making sense of conversations and interactions, and not meeting our relationship partner's need for validation and understanding <br>• Inability to self-reflect or make sense of one's actions |
| **Anxious/ambivalent/ preoccupied** Developed from inconsistent caregiving which confuses the child about what to expect. Traits as adults: <br>• Clingy <br>• Find it hard to trust <br>• Hyper-vigilant about ruptures in relationships | ADHD (combined hyperactive-impulsive presentation) | • Anxiety can lead to presenting with increased sensitivity to conversations <br>• Demand avoidance may look like unwillingness to do what is asked <br>• Inability to read emotional signals can lead to conflict, and then being hyper-vigilant about finding out what led to the rupture in relationship |

*(Continued)*

| INSECURE ATTACHMENT STYLES AND TRAITS IN RELATIONSHIPS | COMMON IN | NEURODIVERSE TRAITS THAT MAY APPEAR AS THESE ATTACHMENT STYLES AND COMPOUND CHALLENGES IN RELATIONSHIPS |
|---|---|---|
| • Misread communication and body language<br>• Feel inadequate<br>• Co-dependent<br>• Partners feel like they can't do enough to make the anxious partner feel secure | | • Unpredictability in ADHD symptoms and stress can cause challenges in forming and maintaining relationships |
| **Disorganized (fearful-anxious-avoidant)**<br>Developed from chaotic or traumatic environment at home, fearing the caregiver, who is unpredictable, and not having a real secure foundation to develop emotionally.<br>• Want to be close, but also need an exit plan<br>• Find it hard to be vulnerable with and trust others<br>• Feel anxious when others want to get close<br>• Fear of rejection and abandonment<br>• Tendency to overlap or prematurely end relationships<br>• Low self-esteem | ADHD (combined hyperactive-impulsive and inattentive presentations) | • Sensory and emotional regulation challenges due to changing biology (for example hormonal fluctuations in neurodivergent women's monthly cycle) or stress<br>• Rejection sensitivity dysphoria<br>• Impulsivity<br>• Fear and anxiety lead to detachment when we sense perceived abandonment<br>• Difficulty respecting or maintaining interpersonal boundaries<br>• Executive functioning challenges (running late, disorganized or stressed due to lack of planning) may add chaos to relationships<br>• Personality differences for those who are medicated or use lifestyle strategies to manage neurodivergence and when these strategies are absent in one's life |

Studies have shown that the neurochemistry of an avoidant differs in the early part of the relationship compared to when they settle into one.[20] Being driven by dopamine, the pursuit colours their sense of excitement and engagement, while their inability to release serotonin and oxytocin as the relationship enters into a steady state can create disconnection and distance, which spells relational drama for their partner. Perhaps this is why so many ADHDers need a feeling of excitement from risk-taking to remain interested in a relationship. The problem becomes two-pronged when we are dealing with a neurochemistry that is prone to both wanting adventure and to sticking to routine, as is the case in the AuDHD experience, when the underlying challenge is a state of restlessness and uncertainty.

What we all want is to be understood and accepted for who we are, to have our emotions validated, our authentic needs met, and to find a place we belong. Is that too much to ask in a relationship? The reality is that neurodiverse relationships have multiple layers of complexity anyway. When you add the significant life transitions of a late diagnosis, starting medication or going through therapy, our relationships can add more stress to our lives, and it can be hard to figure out just what is influencing our behaviours – typical neurodivergent traits, sensory overwhelm, personality disorder, a trauma response, life adversity or . . . perhaps we are just hungry?

Maybe we have become too black and white in our thinking, and too quick to label both ourselves and others, and it has become nearly impossible to form, let alone maintain, a relationship with anyone who's less than perfect in our eyes? With self-awareness and compassion, we all have the capacity for growth and change.

## WHAT DO RELATIONSHIPS MEAN TO YOU?

As someone who is currently taking some time out for quiet self-reflection (and by that, I mean intense self-scrutiny) after having experienced so many relationships that have waxed and waned in my life, I recognize how much work is involved in maintaining a conscious relationship with myself and others. To be good in relationships is a skill you learn; it isn't a natural talent for many of us. However, we can learn about ourselves and heal in relationships through open and honest communication, and reflecting on what our partner mirrors back to us.

Our attitude towards relationships may change throughout our lives, following significant life events such as coming of age, pushing boundaries in our teenage years, leaving home for school or work, falling in love with someone you see as your forever, having children with additional needs or caring for an older family member. And, as we've seen, when you go through a life-changing late diagnosis of ADHD and/or autism.

You will probably look back and realize that the way you showed up in relationships and the choices you made were largely driven by the level of your emotional and mental maturity at the time, as well as pre-conditioned societal beliefs from the culture and circumstances that shaped you. Perhaps you unconsciously repeated unhelpful attachment patterns or reacted in larger-than-expected scale to interactions that ignited rejection sensitivity dysphoria in you. Perhaps you wonder if your parents will ever understand your neurodivergence or mental health diagnosis. Perhaps your diagnosis saved your relationship with your children, because you now understand them more.

The first step in understanding how we show up and impact others in our relationships with them is to take a good look at ourselves and strengthen our self-awareness. This self-knowledge can help us make sense of our behaviours and also those of the people we interact with in our lives. With increasing self-awareness and a better understanding of humanity, you may feel the strong urge to identify unhealthy behaviours and know what you need to work on to become more emotionally mature. From this space, you will better be able to forge stronger, healthier and more lasting relationships with others. However, being more self-aware doesn't necessarily make this stage of our lives any easier, especially if we have a tendency to hyper-fixate on our traits and forget that we are indeed human, with a nervous system that is primed for certain reactions based on the memories from our emotional histories.

In the here and now, it might dawn on you that a seismic mental and emotional shift within you makes it impossible for you to ignore the inevitable changes that need to happen in your current relationships. Some relationships are meant to go the distance with you. These relationships are often built on a foundation of trust, honesty, integrity, mutual desire and commitment to meet both of your emotional needs. However, some relationships just aren't meant to last the course, no matter how hard you try, whether this is due to your or the other person's incompatible vision for the relationship, unmet emotional needs, a build-up of resentment or lack of respect over time.

## UNDERSTANDING YOUR OWN RELATIONSHIP NEEDS

When you have an increased need to be understood, to state your uniqueness, to advocate for your differences, to ask for support and to search for belonging, this will inevitably affect your relationships.

The table below shows a list of the types of relationships that you may evaluate and how you may approach them on your journey.

| RELATION-SHIP TYPE | WHAT IT MEANS TO YOU FOLLOWING A LATE DIAGNOSIS |
| --- | --- |
| With yourself | • Getting to know your authentic self.<br>• Dismantling the old you and way of being, for example quitting unhealthy self-medicating behaviours.<br>• Adopting a healthier lifestyle and a kinder mindset towards yourself.<br>• Going inward: learning your true identity; understanding your needs; re-parenting your inner child (your unconscious mind, which holds onto the emotions, memories and experiences from childhood); attuning to your values; strengthening your sense of self; gaining self-acceptance and self-compassion. |

*(Continued)*

| RELATION-SHIP TYPE | WHAT IT MEANS TO YOU FOLLOWING A LATE DIAGNOSIS |
|---|---|
|  | - Feeling more confident about stating your uniqueness.
- Regress/despair/breakdown while addressing your trauma in therapy.
- Advocating for your differences to family, friends, romantic partners and work.
- Exposure to difficult emotions, learning to regulate them and widen your window of tolerance.
- Radical acceptance of where and who you are, learning to love yourself and show up authentically.
- Designing a life that you love.
- Carving space for self-care and instilling boundaries.
- Post-traumatic growth. |
| Romantic relationships | - Being honest with what you both want out of a romantic relationship: love, companionship, security, passion, belonging, growth, aliveness and so on.
- Determining if you have a shared vision, or if you are willing to meet the other halfway.
- Identifying the strengths in each other that you appreciate.
- Identifying one thing about each other's brain that you'd like to understand better.
- Healing dysfunctional reactions from your autonomic nervous system, and identifying unhealthy patterns and disrupting them; noting your role as well as your partner's in how dysfunctional patterns play out; understanding how your behaviour can create emotional distance and prevent fulfilment; healing from traumatic triggers so you show up as a better version of yourself. |

| RELATION-SHIP TYPE | WHAT IT MEANS TO YOU FOLLOWING A LATE DIAGNOSIS |
|---|---|
| | • Focusing on developing solid foundations by being clear about what you want from the relationship, learning to say no kindly, learning to say yes authentically, and being consistent in your commitment.<br>• Learning to communicate your needs.<br>• Listening and responding with humility and compassion rather than reacting.<br>• Learning your partner's love language and seeing if you are both able and willing to put in the work to love each other in the way you desire and want to be loved.<br>• Learning to be vulnerable.<br>• Identifying if you can and are willing to complement each other's skills in the relationship – for example, one person brings the emotional intelligence and the other brings practical and logistical thinking.<br>• Supporting both of your individual growths on the path to greater emotional fulfilment. |
| Familial relationships | • Gaining awareness of the foundation of your attachment style based on how you were raised in the family environment.<br>• Coming to terms with the relationship you have with your parents, feeling grateful for the love, support and security or feeling angry and hurt for the trauma or neglect.<br>• Hopefully coming to realize that your parents raised you in the ways that they knew, given the resources they had, and accept that even if they couldn't meet your needs, you can heal from the pain, no longer dwell on it, and move on. |

*(Continued)*

| RELATION-SHIP TYPE | WHAT IT MEANS TO YOU FOLLOWING A LATE DIAGNOSIS |
|---|---|
| | • Breaking the cycle of generational trauma by learning to heal your traumatic triggers so you can learn to hold the space for your neurodivergent kids and provide them with validation, emotional support and a sense of belonging that will help them build resilience to life's challenges.<br>• Apologizing to and repairing with your children in moments when you found it hard to provide emotional safety for them.<br>• Adapting your communication style to your child's needs, using clear words and visual prompts to help land a point.<br>• Establishing predictable routines based on interests that provide a sense of security, and sensory-friendly spaces that promote energy recovery.<br>• Seeking professional support to tailor strategies that facilitate secure attachment development for neurodiverse kids. |
| Social relationships | • Understanding the level of social connection you need vs time to recharge from the sensory and social stimulation.<br>• Being intentional about building a community or being part of a support network with like-minded connections.<br>• Reaching out to a community of other ADHDers or autistic individuals with similar experiences, who are committed to finding themselves and supporting each other.<br>• Attending inclusive and accessible events with the neurodiverse community, and being among people who are committed to understanding and acceptance to provide a grounding and reassuring presence beyond the felt sense.<br>• Finding a sense of safety and belonging. |

## STEP 6: EXPECT YOUR RELATIONSHIPS TO CHANGE AND ADAPT

I feel like our collective neurodiverse community sought a diagnosis because we were done with being stuck with the challenges we faced. Being diagnosed with ADHD and autism later in life is like gaining an owner's manual. We become more optimistic about creating a life that we can fall in love with. But the reality is, as we turn on the healing mode on our path to inner transformation, there are going to be bumps along the way and a lot of explaining of the reasons behind our behaviours to the people in our corner. There are going to be times when it will feel more painful to be so conscious of your way of being, because you can no longer hide from it. You are going to be challenged to face the whole of yourself, the parts that everyone loves and the parts that are hard to love.

The changes that are taking place internally within you are going to be felt by those around you – your partner, children, friends, parents and colleagues. You are going to find yourself in a transitionary stage between the person you were in the past and the person you want to become. There may ensue a period of instability ahead, while you renegotiate your needs from the vantage point of your newly acquired knowledge of who you are. This may be met with acceptance and support by your loved ones while you learn about each other's needs, but in relationships that were formed because of an innate habit of self-abandonment, it may also be met with pushback and friction. And when it feels unsettling to deal with conflict, you may now feel an unfamiliar need to instil your own boundaries. This may create yet more friction and may push you into regressing to your old ways of pleasing others. But you will feel probably uncomfortable about this too and wonder who this new person is, the person you're becoming who believes they deserve to be happy and loved, that they deserve to be here. And that they deserve to be safe, even if it is you who have to learn to provide this for yourself.

You can't even resort to the old ways of soothing yourself anymore, now you have a name for the intense pain you feel in your body when you feel unseen, unheard, misunderstood or rejected – rejection sensitivity dysphoria (RSD).

## WHAT TO EXPECT IN THE SHORT-TERM – COPING WITH RSD

Psychologists Geraldine Downey and Scott Feldman introduced the concept of rejection sensitivity dysphoria and how it affects relationships.[21] RSD commonly afflicts ADHDers and autistic individuals, and involves experiencing extreme emotional pain and sensitivity when you perceive what someone else says or does as entailing a rejection of yourself. This often comes from relational or interpersonal triggers, from teasing, criticism, withdrawal of love, respect or approval, or your own inner critic turning against you. The struggle then ensues from the negative overthinking loop that when:

**Externalized** can cause anger outburst, social withdrawal and create relationship problems.
**Internalized** can cause depression, suicide ideation and negative self-talk.

RSD can make us anticipate rejection and do everything in our power to avoid it, from being a people-pleaser and/or perfectionist to becoming a social recluse to avoid embarrassing ourselves socially. This is unsurprising because the pain from feeling rejected and excluded is processed by the same area of the brain that processes physical pain, the dorsal anterior cingulate cortex and the anterior insula, which explains why it can physically hurt when we are rejected.[22]

### The Antidote to RSD

This depends on your neurotype and the source of the RSD episode. Here are some strategies to tackle an intense emotional reaction:

**Stop what you are doing:** if you are with other people, remove yourself to a safe space.

**Reset your autonomic nervous system:** regulate your breathing as your nervous system may be hyper-aroused (angry or stressed) or hypo-aroused (feeling despair or lost). Examples of quick strategies to engage our vagus nerve to restore safety in our bodies include cold therapy (submerging the face in icy water or eating ice lollies), gentle stretching, rocking, hugging or a warm bath or shower.

**Emotional awareness:** witness your emotions without judgement, validate your emotions, and affirm that the difficult thoughts and feelings will pass.

**Give yourself time:** allow yourself time to deal with the emotional flooding and deactivation of your amygdala (your emotional system) and eventually the activation of your frontal lobes (your rational and logical thinking system).

**Restore safety in yourself by seeking glimmers:** reach out and do activities that help you feel safe, connected and happy. For example, connect with a compassionate friend or partner who wants the best for you, spend time in nature, practise mindfulness, yoga or meditation, read a good book, eat nourishing food, or relax with essential oils and soothing music.

**Medication options:** both guanfacine and clonidine have been known to help some ADHDers with RSD, but do consult with a medical professional before making any changes to your medication.

Amid the changes that take place in our lives, autistic individuals may experience 'depression attacks', a serious psychological emergency that can arrive unexpectedly and can be very intense. According to Dr Tony Attwood, a world-renowned clinical psychologist specializing in Asperger syndrome, the triggers are often when one externalizes agitated depression in the form of anger and despair. When autistic individuals experience this emotional implosion, they have a desperate need to end the despair, which can be dangerous for the sufferer.

## How to Support an Autistic Individual During a Depression Attack

Here are some strategies that Dr Attwood recommends for loved ones to support autistic individuals going through this.

| DO | DON'T |
|---|---|
| Stay calm | Interrogate (autistic individuals say, 'I can hear but my brain can't process what people say') |
| Affirm and validate emotions and understand the feelings will go | Move in too close without asking |
| One person to talk to autistic individuals | Try to 'fix' the problem |
| Engage in minimal speech | Use intense eye contact |
| Stay with the person | |
| Encourage engagement in a special interest | |
| Allow time to process intense emotions | |

Attacks of depression often don't last long, and they may require solitude, when the individual affected can take the time to process what's happening, and their thoughts and feelings, before being able to move into an emotionally more balanced state.

## WHAT TO EXPECT IN THE LONG TERM – STEPPING INTO AUTHENTICITY

Once you start to develop self-awareness in the wake of a life-changing diagnosis of ADHD, you can expect the following: growth and transformation. These words can inspire excitement, but in reality, this journey requires a lot of work and staying power.

One day, you're going through the daily motions of life, none the wiser about how your presence affects those around you, and the next, you are catapulted into this state of consciousness. When you've woken up to who you are, it's really hard to unsee this and pretend you're unchanged. You start to examine your relationships through a new lens, and see that the quality of your interactions affects how well you feel in your life. So, if you want to lead a life of fulfilment, you can't get away with not knowing what drives your behaviour and actions.

As Bessel van der Kolk states in *The Body Keeps the Score*, there are two versions of the stories we tell: the version we tell the world, and the version we tell ourselves. The default mode network houses the stories of our self, and this is often over-activated in neurodivergents and those with history of trauma. It's important we recognize this when we do the inner work.

So what stories should you tell yourself? That you are worthy of love, that you're enough, and that when your core wounds are triggered, you can look at yourself and the person who triggered them with compassion, and learn to act from love rather than defiance, withdrawal and anger.

And what about the stories you tell others? If you can learn to express what you feel from the stories you tell yourself, then you will build a bridge rather than a wall between your inner self and the outer world. From this place of self-awareness, accompanied by a sense of agency that is felt inward and expressed outward, your emotional awareness grows, providing fertile soil in which to sow the seeds of a healthy relationship with yourself and others.

However, if you are often in conflict with yourself and your intentions and actions are misaligned with your thoughts and feelings, then you will tend to show up with the parts of yourself at war, causing drama in your life, which inadvertently increases anxiety, depression and anger in your daily interactions.

The world would be such a better place if we were all radically honest with ourselves, to face our truth with courage, show up with vulnerability and compassion in our relationships, and do no harm unto others. When you live your life authentically and freely express yourself, the air feels different. You are also received with more coherence.

---

### What Could Striving for Authenticity Look Like for You?

In the process of getting there, this is what the journey may look like for you.

**Dismantle:** When you find the strength to face your challenges head on and take a long and hard look at your behaviours and what drives them, this will open the way to deconstruct any maladaptive strategies you have.

**Excavate:** Go inward to address the unconscious memories that controlled your reactions, where you'll find both darkness and light. You'll see the stories of fear, grief and anger that give you a distorted lens through which you see the world, and rewrite the narratives for hope, joy and connection. You may stumble at first, but visualize the life you want from hereon and feel into the emotions and thoughts that are associated with the version of yourself that you want to be.

**Rebuild:** After introspection comes action, where you use the lessons you learned from the challenges to help you show up in a new way. You may notice you no longer react as intensely to old triggers. Your behaviour is more deliberate and the people around you will sense an impactful change. From darkness comes a new strength and purpose.

**Emerge:** Show up as your authentic self, becoming more joyful, grateful and resilient to adversity, and prepared to give and receive love. You may radiate a state of peace that makes you magnetic to those on a parallel journey. You may find yourself face to face with experiences that challenge you and which may make you regress at times. It's important to take a step back for introspection and learn to communicate effectively and be open to feedback. Embrace a process of continuous learning and growth.

As you dismantle your old way of being, there's every chance your relationships will grow and thrive from here on, but there are also some that may come to a natural end. It's important that you don't try and do this alone, so seek compassionate connection.

As part of reviewing your relationships after being diagnosed with ADHD, you may find yourself reconsidering your work life, too, which brings us onto Step 7. First, though, I'd like to invite you to start planning now to create the life you want.

## Design the Life You Want

There are many different approaches to designing the life you want. For now, I would like you to reflect on the following prompts:

1. Which people and activities light you up?

2. How could you bring more of these into your life? (For example, through taking up a course or joining a group?)
3. What practical small steps can you take in the short term to achieve this? And in the long term?
4. How can you turn these steps into realistic goals?
5. What discussions might you have with those close to you about making changes that allow you to pursue these goals?
6. Is there anyone who could mentor you or who inspires you as a role model?

# Step 7:
# Navigate Your Neurodiversity at Work

'Neurodiversity' refers to the diversity of the human mind, the way we think, learn, process information, feel and act in the world. It includes all humans on earth. As members of society with useful contributions to make, neurodivergents have a right to equality and to feel that our unique insights and strengths are acknowledged, respected and valued. This applies to our role in the workplace.

This is why the neurodiversity movement is focused on displacing the medical model of disability. Instead of seeing a neurodivergent individual as impaired and in need of being fixed, the movement subscribes to the social model of disability, where the social barriers created through the way society is organized are the reasons neurodivergents struggle to fit in. The idea is that when we support neurodivergents with their needs, we remove the barriers created by society and enable these individuals to harness their strengths and fulfil their potential.

In order to harness our strengths, we need to get to the bottom of why we have difficulties fitting in in the first place and find the right tools for each individual. However, talking about our difference can have the unintended effect of marginalizing us further. This is why, while it's important to celebrate our differences, I feel the way to create a more effective culture is to help everyone understand that many of the areas that neurodivergents find challenging are shared by those who do not identify as a neurodivergent. When we create a workplace that is accessible to all minds, everyone benefits.

What makes it complex to know how to support neurodivergents is that each of us will have different areas that we find easy and challenging, as neurodivergence isn't a one-size-fits-all approach. Our lives are shaped by our unique neurological wiring, and it starts with creating a space for individuals to share their own stories and define their own realities.

What makes neurodivergents happy and content in their jobs? I deeply believe that in order to answer this question, we need to understand why work is so important to neurodivergents. Why do some of us autistic and/or ADHDers find it hard to stop working? Why do some of us find it hard to start? Why is it so important that we do the kind of work that gives us an outlet for our creativity, single focus, special interest, search for deeper meaning and purpose, or innate expression?

In Step 7 of the ADHD iceberg, we are going to dive into neurodiversity in the workplace and consider the challenges and barriers that ADHDers can face there – from the interview stage to coping with the demands of the working environment and interacting with colleagues. We'll be also touching upon the feelings of stigma and shame that we can often face around our approach to work. And I'll be offering guidance on how to bridge the empathy gap between employers and their neurodiverse employees, as well as what to do if you find yourself in a non-supportive working environment.

Let's roll up our sleeves and get down to business!

THE SEARCH FOR MEANINGFUL WORK

As an autistic ADHDer who has worked in 16 different industries, I spent what feels like decades searching for the kind of work that truly lights me up. Having worked in everything from academia, science research, pharmaceuticals, writing and travel journalism, communications, commercial modelling, acting, translation, interpreting, tutoring, retail, food and beverage, hospitality and soft furnishings, to creating a social impact company, becoming a keynote speaker, and a neurodiversity trainer and consultant, I can confirm that my most authentic motivation isn't about money, prestige nor status. It may sound ridiculous, but it is more important for me to honour my need for autonomy, honesty, integrity, creative expression and intellectual fulfilment, as well as being able to live to my values.

When I got diagnosed with ADHD and found out about the interest-based nervous system that is typical for ADHDers and autistic individuals, it made so much sense. We are guided by what is interesting, challenging, novel, urgent and passionate to us. It was very hard for me to light up when I had a job that didn't have any of these elements, no matter how hard I tried. It was especially hard when I didn't know what I was doing and instructions were unclear, and when my anxiety about not meeting expectations worsened into a panic attack during one of my highest paid contract roles.

Rather than merely explaining our way of being via neurological differences such as monotropism or special interests, or via the traumatized lens of needing to derive our entire self-esteem from our work, I believe that when we do the kind of work that lights us up, we move into a flow state – it is as though we are a city at night with every street lamp lighting up in succession, illuminating a soothing glow within. In this state, every part of us feels coherent and we connect with inner peace and contentment. It recharges our batteries. Perhaps this peace is what we all try to find externally through various means, substances or activities, if we haven't yet found a way to channel this within ourselves.

Now imagine if this type of work becomes something the world needs and that others would pay you for? And you keep at it day in and day out because your interest in this area takes you so deep and so wide in your level of knowledge to land at the top of your chosen industry? Imagine if your identity presents a well-lit path that supports your success?

When I finally understood my unique neurotype, it felt like I could put an end to my restless exploration for a role that fulfilled me, as I accepted that I have always needed to create my own place in the world of work. When I made peace with being self-employed, I discovered just how common it was for neurodivergents to work for themselves (20–35 per cent are freelancers) and to be entrepreneurs (55 per cent), and how many are unemployed (30–40 per cent) due to the challenges of fitting in.

This seals the importance of helping neurodivergents access the potential within them and channelling this into work that lights them up. Do they enjoy their work and do they feel like they can fulfil their potential in that environment? When given opportunities to upskill and take their interests and depth of knowledge far into the pinnacle of their career, many neurodivergents find themselves in leadership positions. Indeed, research has found that 45 per cent of C-level executives (CEOs, CFOs, COOs) and 32 per cent of senior management self-identify as neurodivergents.[1] Besides this, given the fact that 76 per cent of employees say they are more likely to stay in a company that prioritizes training opportunities means that we are looking at a population, neurodivergent or not, who are looking for a career that fulfils their individual expression, interest, and dare I say it, purpose.

### What Does Meaningful Work Look Like for You?

Does your work light you up and are you fulfilling your potential? To find some answers, here are some questions to reflect upon:

1. Do I like the work I am doing?
2. Am I in the best place that supports my career and individual growth?
3. Do I feel safe here to express myself without the fear of repercussion?
4. Can I get the support I need to tap into my strengths here?

## REVIEWING YOUR WORK LIFE AFTER YOUR DIAGNOSIS

At a time when so many neurodivergents are grappling with a late diagnosis or are contemplating one (and are therefore self-identified), 'disclosure' needs to be handled with sensitivity because there's often many competing priorities in their minds.

In an ideal world, when we get a diagnosis, we will have been in a company for a while and have good rapport with our manager, so opening up about our neurodivergence is not an immediate concern. However, according to research by the Institution of Occupational Safety and Health (IOSH), the reality is that at least 70 per cent of neurodivergents haven't mentioned this to their manager or human resources (HR) department.[2]

In my experience, many neurodivergents, and especially those who are self-identified, bottle up their neurodivergence until they get to a point where it's blurted out at a performance review or at the point of dismissal – where they are in a state of fight-or-flight.[3] It then becomes a little awkward for everyone. The neurodivergent individual is now being seen as making excuses, while the managers are put in a tricky place of needing to find legal advice around how to sensitively handle the situation to avoid the situation being escalated to an employment tribunal.

To truly make a difference, we need to create a workplace environment where people *want* to stay. Especially for a neurodivergent, the need to feel safe, understood and accepted is paramount, as is to feel they belong.

There are many companies that are progressive on this front. They have created a neurodiversity policy in their diversity, equity and inclusion company policies, carried out company-wide awareness and manager's training, provided reasonable adjustments, formed employee resource groups, and regularly host webinars and get-togethers to foster a neuroinclusive culture. However, unfortunately many others, if not the majority of companies, are lagging behind due to the lack of intention or funding for these efforts.

And while we are on the subject, neurodivergents in unsafe work cultures wrestle with the fear of being misunderstood and unsupported, anxiety around stigma, stress, burnout and low moods. This ultimately affects their productivity and performance, culminating in an intention to leave the company and start anew elsewhere. This demotivation is reflected in neurodivergents' mental wellbeing, which is at a very low score at work of 2.02.[4]

## COMMON CHALLENGES AND BARRIERS

Let's look at some common challenges faced by members of our community at work – from access barriers at the interview stage to stepping through the company's door and participating in its daily activities.

Many of the challenges can be found in the nature of the job, as areas such as managing professional relationships, socio-communication differences, and the nature of the task itself can become a source of misunderstanding and confusion.

Many neurodivergents think that knowing about their way of being has helped them advocate for whatever challenges they need support with. While this is true and can be helpful, often, we need to ask ourselves how being more aware of these challenges actually makes us feel, and how our managers and colleagues will receive this information.

**Reflection**
Take a moment now to consider this list. Does anything on it strike a chord with you? What changes or support might help?

| CHALLENGES FOR NEURO-DIVERGENTS | WHAT THIS LOOKS LIKE |
| --- | --- |
| Interview | • Inaccessible way of relaying information<br>• Speaking before thinking of the consequences<br>• Answering open-ended interview questions by going off on a tangent<br>• Difficulty performing social niceties such as small talk and eye contact, which lead to misunderstanding |

| CHALLENGES FOR NEURO-DIVERGENTS | WHAT THIS LOOKS LIKE |
|---|---|
| Manager | • Micromanagement (lack of autonomy)<br>• Lack of compassion and understanding<br>• Difficulty implementing boundaries<br>• Unclear expectations and communication<br>• Lack of accountability<br>• Insistence of standard working norms, for example working times, being seen in the office, no remote working option<br>• Not implementing reasonable adjustments, or implementing them but not considering it during performance review |
| Professional relationships | • Social group situations cause social anxiety<br>• Difficulty understanding how to interact in a socially-accepted way<br>• Rejection sensitivity dysphoria from interactions<br>• Burnout |
| Communication | • Not understanding jokes and sarcasm (especially autistic or AuDHDers)<br>• Delay in processing information leading to difficulty following conversations<br>• Difficulty retaining information relayed in a verbal way |
| The work itself caused by executive function difficulties and mental health | • Productivity<br>• Organizing workload<br>• Creating structure<br>• Managing distractions<br>• Keeping track of things that need a follow up<br>• Admin tasks<br>• Imposing deadlines<br>• Working according to a neurotypical mode of working and output<br>• Burnout |

*(Continued)*

| CHALLENGES FOR NEURO-DIVERGENTS | WHAT THIS LOOKS LIKE |
|---|---|
| Meetings | • Having back-to-back meetings<br>• Having to sit down all day<br>• Finding it hard to remember what was said<br>• Exhaustion from dealing with too many people<br>• Keeping up with standard workplace norms |
| Mental health | • Anxiety<br>• Panic attacks<br>• Burnout |
| Work doesn't harness individual's strengths and interest | • Work that does not fulfil one's interest, passion or purpose<br>• Lack of career development and opportunity to upskill |
| Self-advocacy | • Uncertainty around how neurodivergence will be received due to stigma<br>• Difficulty receiving reasonable adjustment<br>• Not knowing what support is available and needed<br>• Being ignored by manager |

## TURNING SHAME INTO STRENGTH

Once we have a name to put to our challenges, this can often become a point of focus, along with the shame that is uncovered by such awareness. We may even forget how to do the things we once knew in the name of 'executive dysfunction', undoing all the coping strategies we'd learned over decades of living. One of the ways I'd learned to cope with this renewed understanding of my neurodivergent identity is to uncover the reason behind the source of my shame and reframe this based on my individual reality so I can stop chastising myself.

As you'll have gleaned from the Steps before this, our lived experience of neurodivergence is far more nuanced than either the 'superpower' or 'disability' tropes suggest. It's a complex interplay of strengths and challenges, triumphs and struggles all unfolding within the context of a society that's still learning how to embrace and support neurological diversity.

Beyond the whimsical surface of 'celebrating neurodiversity', there's a humane explanation of a step-by-step process that makes us. Not everyone is going to resonate with all the traits within the labels of ADHD and co-occurring conditions such as autism, and this is why it remains shrouded in mystery as we process the labels within ourselves.

For example, the next time you find yourself saying something along the lines of, 'Oh, my ADHD makes me stay up late at night due to delayed sleep phase syndrome and therefore makes me turn up late at work', you should be aware that there may well be other interacting factors in your life that are making sleep even more elusive for you at this time, such as menopause symptoms, chronic stress, caring responsibilities or stimulants. If this is the case, then there are some very real biological changes that are happening inside you that deserve your compassion and attention.

Understanding a very important fact can help to reframe any potential shame around our work productivity and output: that a neurodivergent mind works in wondrous ways that diverge from what society considers as the norm. By the norm here, I'm referring to the standard systems, processes and results that are considered the 'way people do things here', which don't always work for a divergent mind. When we can learn to accept that we have unique ways of thinking, learning and processing information, and feel that we are not lesser than, just different, we will be able to be kinder to ourselves, and silence the harsh inner critic that has been our companion for far too long.

The reality is that neurodivergents want to be understood, accepted and supported with our challenges, and we want to work with our strengths because deep down, we know that the genius within our mind is worth its weight in gold, if only we have a reliable way of channelling it into the world!

## How We Can Reframe Shame into Strength?

| MYTHS ABOUT ADHD OR AUDHD TRAITS AS SEEN FROM THE OUTSIDE | REALITY AND AFFIRMATIONS |
|---|---|
| I am lazy | - I have a different way of prioritizing tasks, which means that some tasks will induce me into action and some just won't get my brain ticking no matter how hard I try! If I know what my strengths are, then I can focus on them, and get support for things that I find challenging.<br>- There is a lot going on in my head that can cause me to feel too immobilized and paralysed to act.<br>- I am trying to recover from a long time spent in hyper-focus, as all my energy was used to create a kind of tunnel vision which now leaves me feeling depleted. |
| I am procrastinating on this, why can't I just get motivated? | - There are certain times of the day when my brain comes to life, and when I miss that window, I'll have to wait for tomorrow.<br>- I have imposter syndrome around this project and I worry that if I don't create my best work ever, I will be judged. |
|  | - I am picking up on nuances around an idea that help me create a better solution to the problem I'm solving, and it takes time for me to process what this means to the bigger picture. |

| MYTHS ABOUT ADHD OR AUDHD TRAITS AS SEEN FROM THE OUTSIDE | REALITY AND AFFIRMATIONS |
|---|---|
| I am so disorganized and chaotic | • There are multiple ideas swirling in my head. If I'm able to tap into the brilliance, I'll be unstoppable.<br>• I am able to see patterns and spot connections within the problem I am trying to solve – there's method in my madness! |
| I am a loner | • I often come up with the best inspirations when I'm alone and have time to reflect. This sparks creativity and innovation.<br>• I find people loud and unpredictable, and while I like one-to-one interaction, I can find groups overstimulating and need to recover in solitude. |
| I don't hold eye contact and can have a blank expression at times, which can be tough when it comes to making friends | • I am still absorbing and processing the information relayed to me and I have a different way of empathizing with others. Even when I appear vacant on the surface, I feel what others feel intensely in my body even if I may not show it in my facial expressions. |
| I tend to disrupt people in mid conversation | • I need to convey what I'm thinking or I'll forget! |

## BECOMING MORE AWARE OF ATTITUDES AT WORK

While you are coming to terms with your unique neurodivergent mind, you also need to suss out what your workplace's understanding is around neurodiversity. Below is a checklist to help you assess their readiness and/or ability to support you.

- Notice how your colleagues and manager respond when the conversation is steered towards ADHD and/or autism, the rise in diagnoses and neurodiversity.
- Does your workplace culture feel safe?
- Do you feel free to contribute ideas in your team without the fear of repercussions?
- How is your rapport with your manager and the rest of the team?
- Do you have a balanced view of your neurodivergence from a position of its strengths and challenges?
- Has your workplace had a neurodiversity awareness session that is framed via a mission to work together?
- Does your workplace recognize the strengths in diversity of thought?
- Does a clear workplace needs assessment pathway exist to identify reasonable adjustments?

If you decide to open up about your neurodiversity to your colleagues, it matters how you talk about it. By focusing too much on your challenges, you are essentially singling yourself out as different or lesser than, which can create a sense of separation from the rest of the team. For example, early on in my journey, I came across a coach who taught people to communicate their ADHD or autism via the pathologized and medicalized model often seen in healthcare, which really wasn't helpful. And time and time again when managers come to me looking for support, this shows me how we can't risk shooting ourselves in the foot before we even have the chance to prove ourselves. So please let's not invite more infantilization for conditions like ADHD and AuDHD, which are already historically burdened with stigma.

On the other hand, I am amazed and impressed by those who do a good job at opening up about their neurodivergence and where it is received with understanding and compassion. When this happens, it's often the result of many of the following stars being aligned – self-empowered communication, good rapport with the manager and team, humour as an inherent personality trait in the neurodivergent individual, ability to connect with others, a compassionate and supportive line manager, and a neurodiversity-aware HR team. Often, these empowered neurodivergents may even go on to form employee resource groups, which can be powerful entities that enable other like-minded people in the company to come together in a community.

I'm not saying the prospect ahead is always rosy, but if you get your self-advocacy right to begin with, you will be starting off on a much better footing.

## HOW TO COMMUNICATE YOUR NEEDS TO YOUR COLLEAGUES

So how do you communicate your neurodivergence in ways that will give you the best chance of success? It's a good idea to consider whether you will need an ally at any conversation about it with your line manager or HR team. This will depend in part on the sort of answers you came up with earlier about attitudes in your workplace and whether you feel safe and understood there. If you need an ally, find one who is ideally in a position of influence and power, and who also knows the quality of your work.

Here are some prompts to help you prepare for your conversation around reasonable adjustments:

- Focus on the strengths you bring to your job and what they originally saw in you that led to you being hired.
- Find a common purpose in terms of what you and your company both want to achieve, and start exploring solutions that will allow you both to achieve that goal.
- Talk about your neurodivergence from the balanced total of your strengths and needs – but not skewed too heavily on the needs.
- Be your own cheerleader while explaining what challenges are creating barriers for you to achieve your best results, for example in your day-to-day tasks or the organization's ways of working.
- Suggest specific adjustments that would make your work life easier, for example noise-cancelling headphones, flexible working hours or administrative support. Be as specific as possible.
- Come prepared with a clear and concise explanation of how your requested adjustments will help you thrive in your role.
- Be prepared to collaborate and co-create solutions. Your employer might have suggestions or alternatives you haven't considered. Be willing to engage in dialogue and discuss alternative ways of working that suit everyone involved.
- Agree on a set of adjustments and a trial period, where you and your line manager or HR department can review the situation at a specified date in the near future.
- Ask for a check-in as you get used to the adjustments to see if they work for you.

It's important that you ask for understanding as you transition into this space of working to your strengths and being supported for your needs, as more than likely, there'll be teething issues for no other reason than this is an area that many companies are only now navigating for the first time.

As you transition into having some adjustments and workplace support, it can feel as though you are finally getting through and being heard. It's important for your manager to know that it'll take you time to find out what works and what doesn't, so you'll need to manage their expectations and they shouldn't expect you to fly right away! Many neurodivergents say that when they receive reasonable adjustments tailored to them and they feel understood by management and their colleagues, it gives them the permission to thrive.

## NAVIGATING PERFORMANCE FEEDBACK

Of all the places where members of the neurodivergent community can potentially put our foot in our mouth at work, the annual performance review is the one we can't always resist. The anxiety that can accompany a looming performance review may heighten our rejection sensitivity dysphoria (RSD, see page 212) and enhance our inner critic before we even sit down and start the process.

Afterwards, we feel that points raised in the performance review were unjustified, given the fact that we are often evaluated on our abilities to carry out and achieve a desired result without the support we need to do so. I've often heard from neurodivergent employees who feel misunderstood as they are perceived to perform poorly when the reason they struggle in the first place is due to the organization's insistence on following systems and processes that are inaccessible to their way of thinking, learning and processing styles, as well as unclear expectations, communication differences, being made to work with their challenges without support, and much more.

Managers should also consider if their feedback is unintentionally biased or if the concerns that they raise can be accommodated by the individual whose performance is being reviewed. Without a thorough understanding of how to harness our strengths and the type of support we need for our challenges, no matter how enthusiastic we are at our jobs to begin with, the frustration of not being supported at work can be followed by the sinking feeling of inadequacy over time. In an ideal world, we would be evaluated based on our strengths and the things that we know deep down we can do better than anyone else.

While we know that work appraisals like performance reviews are necessary, in reality, neurodivergent or not, no one likes to receive critical feedback. It takes us straight into our emotional brain, primed to defend or argue our way out of things.

The antidote for the RSD we ADHDers often experience is positive feedback, which is why I would always advise managers and colleagues to lead with the good feedback. Positive feedback activates a sense of recognition responsive euphoria (RRE), a term I first heard from Dr Ned Hallowell, an ADHD expert, psychiatrist and renowned author. While negative feedback can be painful, no matter how tactfully delivered, RRE has the opposite effect, giving us a good boost and strengthening our resilience. RRE delivers a meaningful and powerful zing of energy and esteem with every word of encouragement, praise or approval we receive.

The power of sincere and positive acknowledgement of our strengths and light can propel us to do great work and even go on to attain wonderful accomplishments. Some ADHDers or autistic individuals have gone on to forge an entire career based on this sort of praise – you know who you are!

## WHAT DOES A SUPPORTIVE WORK ENVIRONMENT LOOK LIKE?

Underneath all the corporate HR speak, there needs to be a very human understanding of our neurodiverse experiences, which shows in the way we and our colleagues communicate, interact and empathize with one another. A supportive workplace for neurodiversity has a work culture that embraces and values a diversity of thought and levels the playing field for all employees so they can utilize their strengths. The table below shows what a supportive environment that makes a difference to neurodivergents might look like in practice. While this sounds like a workplace that anyone would value, these strategies will especially benefit neurodivergent employees who have specific needs around accessibility and mental health.

# STEP 7: NAVIGATE YOUR NEURODIVERSITY AT WORK

| COMMON WORKPLACE FEEDBACK | HOW WE MIGHT INTERPRET IT | WHAT INCLUSIVE WORKPLACE FEEDBACK LOOKS LIKE INSTEAD |
|---|---|---|
| The team and I realized you don't join our after-work socials and therefore it's extremely hard to suss out what you're like as a person. | The entire team hates me, I don't belong here, and I don't know if I want to stay in this team. | Hey, I've noticed that you don't often join us for after-work socials. What would be your preference in terms of ways to connect with the team and understand each other's way of working and quirks? |
| The report was meant to be submitted by Thursday. I know you're juggling a lot at the moment, but that deadline was crucial. | I find it really hard to juggle multiple projects simultaneously, and the reason I missed the deadline on that report was because it took me time to switch gears from one task to another. I really need to have dedicated time to focus on one project at a time, and some time to transition to the next project. | Your report was due at end of day Thursday, but it was submitted on Friday. We need to ensure timely submissions as this affects the project as a whole. In the future, what do you need to help you complete it in a timely manner? |
| A senior colleague told me that they felt disrespected when you interrupted the team meeting and gave them an earful of what you thought they could do better. | But I needed to say it, otherwise I would forget. I was only saying what I thought was glaringly obvious. There were typos all over that report and I was only concerned about the quality. If I came across rude, it was because I care about the end result. I often receive feedback for my writing, so why should a senior colleague have special treatment? | I noticed you have a very straightforward way of communicating that can come across as a little blunt to those around you. I think if people understand that you are just stating facts, they would be less likely to take offence. Perhaps we can hold a neurodiversity awareness session to help the team understand? |

*(Continued)*

| COMMON WORKPLACE FEEDBACK | HOW WE MIGHT INTERPRET IT | WHAT INCLUSIVE WORKPLACE FEEDBACK LOOKS LIKE INSTEAD |
|---|---|---|
| It doesn't look good on you and the rest of the team when you walk in at 10am, while most people are at their desk by 9am. | Oh no, it's happening again. No matter how hard I try, I seem to always end up being late in the morning. My brain doesn't switch on until 10am anyway, so it's pointless to get me in at 9am, as this means I'll lose an extra hour of sleep and will struggle with my energy and concentration levels. | I noticed you tend to turn up at 10am most days. I'm okay with this as long as it doesn't affect your productivity and you make up for the hours in your own time. What working hours would suit you in terms of your energy and concentration cycles? We can think of how to make this work for you, as long as this works for the team's project timeline. |
| Your report doesn't seem to contain what we discussed at the meeting. | I couldn't process and capture everything that was said in time, so it would help if I had written instructions and a check-in afterwards. | I noticed some of the things we discussed didn't make it into the report. Do you need any follow up instructions or visual aid to help you with understanding the aim of the task? |
| You started off in this role very enthusiastic and gradually seem to have lost that passion; now you seem demotivated. | They can tell I've lost my mojo. I can't seem to get excited about this project and have asked to be put on a different project but my request seems to be ignored. | I wanted to check in to see how you're doing. You seem a little distracted and I would love to talk about how I can support you to get you back on track. |

## A Neurodiversity-supportive Workplace

| AIM | MEASURES TAKEN |
|---|---|
| Psychological safety, sense of belonging and connection | • Company-wide training of neurodiversity to promote understanding and empathy, reduce stigma, address biases and support employees who are neurodivergent or have children who are.<br>• Management trained to support neurodivergent individuals, providing clear expectations and instructions, accountability, regular constructive feedback and honest and transparent communication to avoid ambiguity and reduce anxiety.<br>• Forming employee neurodiversity resource groups or peer support networks where neurodivergents can connect in judgement-free spaces, share their stories and provide support for each other. |
| Accessible work and neurodivergent-friendly environment | • Tailored reasonable adjustments based on specific needs of neurodivergents, for example workplace adjustments, coaching and task support, alternative communication methods and ways of working.<br>• Flexibility in work hours, remote working options, ways of working to support neurodivergent employees to manage their routines, sensory sensitivities and any other specific needs.<br>• Designing sensory-friendly workspaces including noise-cancelling headphones, adjustable lighting and temperature, and quiet areas to work. |

*(Continued)*

| AIM | MEASURES TAKEN |
|---|---|
| Mental wellbeing | • Compassionate leadership in managers who use their power and influence to prevent the struggles of others, empower others to succeed and enable autonomy.<br>• Managers who regularly seek two-way feedback from neurodivergent employees to understand their experiences, identify areas for improvement, and make necessary adjustments to support their success in the workplace.<br>• A workplace culture that values work–life balance, modelled by senior leaders and colleagues.<br>• Offering wellness programmes and resources such as employee assistance programmes that focus on mental health, stress management and self-care to promote overall wellbeing for all. |
| Career development based on interests, strengths and purpose | • Providing equal opportunities for professional growth, to upskill and curate their roles, tools, training and professional development for all.<br>• Supporting neurodivergent employees with mentors, coaches or sponsors who represent them in meetings that they don't have access to and which enable them to advance in their careers. |

## HOW TO INTEGRATE OUR DIVERSE IDENTITIES IN THE WORKPLACE

In fact, the starter list mentioned in the table will only take us so far in creating the ideal workplace, because there are of course nuances in our neurodiverse experiences. All this means is that we will each have different needs. However, this makes it a very complex exercise when management is trying to spot a neurodivergent in the wild and even more complex when they're trying to figure out what type of support will enhance that individual's productivity and mental health.

One of the biggest reasons for this challenge is that many companies are unaware that if they deliver neurodiversity training without a true understanding of our realities, this can impact individuals who come from diverse identities in ways that aren't always supportive. Often, companies are like mini ecosystems made up of multicultural people who come from different backgrounds and life circumstances. Alongside this, senior leadership will greatly influence the workplace vibe, its norms, culture, purpose and intention. All day long, interactions occur between us and our colleagues, our managers and their managers. Now imagine the challenges in these interactions if we talk about neurodiversity as a one-size-fits-all approach.

As we saw in Steps 3 and 4, in the real world, our neurodiverse experience is a complex interplay between the genes we've inherited and the environment to which we've been exposed since our time in the womb. Our brains, biochemistry, personalities, motivations, physical, mental and emotional needs are influenced by our beginnings, cultural and racial norms, socialization (how our societies shape us by condoning what's acceptable and the ways in which they reject the unacceptable), social class status, and our current life circumstances. The degree of heterogeneity, the *diversity in diversity*, will mean that our unique neurodivergent needs will differ from others around us in the neurodiverse community.

In order for efforts to support neurodiverse individuals at work to truly make a difference in terms of our productivity, achievement and happiness, we need to link these efforts to our life contexts. We cannot look at neurodiversity as an isolated identity.

Under the Equality Act 2010 in the UK, there are nine protected categories for which any form of unfair treatment or discriminatory behaviour is unacceptable and unlawful. These are:

- Age
- Disability
- Gender reassignment

- Marriage and civil partnership
- Pregnancy and maternity
- Race
- Religion or belief
- Sex
- Sexual orientation

Neurodiversity and mental health fall within the disability bracket, which characterizes a physical or mental impairment that significantly affects an individual's ability to perform normal daily tasks. Nevertheless, more companies are moving away from seeing neurodiversity as 'disability' per se; for example, autism and ADHD are increasingly seen as ways of being, not 'disorders' as such. Rather, it's how these neurodiversities are perceived by others or the barriers created by society that can make them appear different.

If you look at the different identities and life circumstances that make up the protected characteristics in the list above, these are all experienced by neurodivergent people too. Men, women, non-binary individuals, LGBTQIA, people of the global majority, Muslims, Buddhists, Christians, Hindus, pregnant women, single people, mothers, fathers, parents, or not . . . many neurodivergents are all of these things. As you've learned in Step 4, there are notable parallels between neurodivergents and intersectional identities – both face challenges, biases and discrimination in a society that is shaped to give privilege to a particular dominant identity. For neurodivergents who also identify with intersectionality, this challenge is compounded mentally, emotionally and physically.

As many of our challenges become more pronounced during life transitions, we are going to need more understanding and support while we find our way. It's important for managers and colleagues to recognize the importance of bringing a humane and empathetic lens to their interactions with us, and to see that each individual is unique and to adapt the support on offer to our unique needs.

This is not to say that because we may need additional support, we are in any respect lesser than our counterparts. Everything that we are and we have experienced during the course of our lives gives us unique insights, problem-solving skills, resilience, wisdom, creativity and leadership skills, all of which can contribute to greater success for the modern workplace that increasingly values original and innovative thought. This is why there needs to be neurodiversity training and support in workplaces through an intersectional lens, where every neurodivergent is recognized for their multi-layered identity and experiences, beyond just their neurodivergent traits.

As for how to integrate our different life contexts in the workplace, how about creating a person-centred approach to inclusion?

| A PERSON-CENTRED APPROACH TO WORKPLACE INCLUSION ||
|---|---|
| Respect individual experiences | Every neurodivergent individual has unique experiences, strengths and challenges that shape their life journey. For example, a neurodivergent person will have more significant and specific needs during big life transitions such as divorce, menopause, pregnancy or parenthood, and would appreciate tailored adjustments in their day to day, during the transition back to work, and support in their mental health. |
| Remove stigma | Intersectional neurodivergents may have endured societal prejudices and discrimination. For example, if a neurodivergent employee is also a person of colour, there may be unconscious bias at their performance review or this may affect their chances of being considered for promotion. |
| Emphasize empathy | Understanding the frustrations, difficulties and triumphs that neurodivergents have endured can foster a more empathetic workplace. |

*(Continued)*

| A PERSON-CENTRED APPROACH TO WORKPLACE INCLUSION ||
|---|---|
| Promote accessibility | Accessibility measures shouldn't only be a reaction to an existing struggle. By considering the myriad challenges neurodivergent individuals have faced, we can proactively create accessible environments that reduce potential barriers. For example, for a parent of a neurodivergent child, there is a greater need for flexibility and understanding around how and when they can work best, and to be given the opportunity and support for career advancement. |
| Advocate for resources | Understanding the challenges neurodivergent individuals have endured can help inform efforts to secure the resources needed for inclusion – from specialized support and mental health resources, accessibility tools, understanding in navigating social situations or tools to support working parents with neurodivergence parenting experts. |
| Increase representation | It's vital for diverse identities to be represented in peer support networks, employee resource groups, teams and leadership positions to create an inclusive, empowered and supportive workforce. |
| Include in decision-making | Ensuring neurodivergent individuals from diverse identities are included in decisions that affect their work lives will ensure their specific needs and experiences are considered from the start. |

When we receive the support that enables us to do our best work, this brings with it a budding sense of freedom – the agency to be our authentic selves and thrive.

If workplace cultures could start to recognize that, essentially, we are all different, and through these differences we're actually more alike than we are unalike, I think we will be primed for a new and improved way of doing things and talking about mental health and brain differences.

## MY WORKPLACE DOESN'T OFFER SUPPORT – NOW WHAT?

It's all very well talking about ideal scenarios, but if you're navigating a late diagnosis of ADHD or AuDHD and find yourself metaphorically stranded on an island within your workplace, with no available support network to turn to, what do you do? How do you go looking for support where there isn't an obvious place to turn?

Well, first of all I would gauge the atmosphere, and see if the workplace environment feels like a safe one in which to talk about your neurodivergence. I say this with the best of intentions, because while some workplaces are often very open to the idea of creating an employee resource group for those with neurodivergence for example, many more may still hold prejudices about these sorts of issues.

The first place you would usually go is your line manager. However, this depends on two things: your rapport with them and if you think they have your back. If you feel comfortable about opening up to them, then use the prompts I set out for you in 'How to Communicate Your Needs to Your Colleagues' on page 231. Your line manager will usually go to HR, who will hopefully have a pathway of support in place, which may involve occupational health and conducting a workplace needs assessment to kickstart your request for reasonable adjustments.

If you feel you need to override your line manager, check your company's HR policy to see if they have a policy for neurodiversity and if they reference the Equality Act 2010 (if in the UK). At the very least, your place of work should have a mental health policy or an employee assistance programme whereby you can request to speak to a therapist or a coach for guidance and support.

Here are some suggestions of what you can do to seek support and adjustments:

- Look after your mental health first and foremost to give yourself the best chance of showing up at work.
- Consider seeking professional support from a workplace neurodiversity trainer and consultant on how to broach this subject and open up to your employer about your support needs.
- If you feel safe to open up to members of your workplace, consider starting a conversation with your HR department about the challenges you face with your neurodivergence and your need for support. Talk to them about how supportive networks and adjustments can make a positive impact on employee wellbeing and retention, citing the best practices of other companies or their competitors in the same industry that are leading in championing neurodiversity.[5]
- Suggest neurodiversity awareness training to HR or management, to activate a company-wide change in understanding neurodivergence. This initiative can help colleagues understand both the strengths and challenges of working with neurodivergence, how to embrace working with neurodivergent colleagues, and instil a sense of psychological safety for them.
- Follow up with management training on neurodiversity to equip line managers with the tools and resources to support their neurodivergent colleagues and instil a sense of safety in the team.
- Look for external resources and other online support networks that may provide guidance, strategies and a sense of community for others who are going through similar challenges.
- Test the waters with colleagues about neurodivergence, and see what they say. If you are able to find a group of like-minded people who share your experience, go and talk to HR together about considering starting an employee support group for neurodiversity together to break down stigma, share experiences and strategies, and support each other in navigating work-related challenges.

## What Would Help You to Shine at Work?

If you would like to talk to your manager or HR about making changes to support you, it pays to be prepared. Take a moment now to consider the following points as succinctly and objectively as you can.

1. In which areas are you struggling? Why do you think this is?
2. What could your workplace do to support you on a day-to-day basis?
3. In which areas are you succeeding? Why do you think this is?
4. What are your skills?
5. What goals do you have that you would like to fulfil? (Keep these SMART: specific, measurable, attainable, relevant and time-based.)
6. What opportunities or additional support might you need to help you achieve these? In what ways do you and your employer stand to benefit?

## Create Your Own Employee Resource Group

By creating an employee resource group (ERG), you will be able to mobilize the intention of a group of people who are not only looking for support but keen on creating a positive cultural change around neurodiversity in your workplace.[6]

You may also find that it is a good idea to combine your diversity and support efforts with other ERGs to form intersectional ERGs, which can create more meaningful support for intersectional neurodivergents. The following is the case for creating an intersectional ERG that you can show your HR and management team:

**Celebrates diversity and inclusion:** These groups bring together individuals from different backgrounds, identities and experiences, creating a workplace culture that values diversity and inclusion.

**Supports you and others like you:** They provide a platform for underrepresented and marginalized employees, including yourself, to speak up, share your perspectives, and advocate for your needs within the organization.

**Learning and growing together:** Through various activities and discussions, these groups help you and your colleagues learn about different identities, experiences and challenges, fostering awareness and understanding.

**Building a strong community:** Being part of these groups gives you a sense of community and belonging, especially when you feel isolated or marginalized at work. It's a safe space where you can all connect, support each other and share your experiences.

**Opportunities for development:** These groups offer chances for professional growth, mentorship, networking and career advancement, helping you improve your skills and build relationships within the organization.

**Fuelling innovation and creativity:** By bringing diverse perspectives together, these groups spark innovation, creativity and problem-solving, enhancing your collective impact within the organization.

**Caring for your wellbeing:** The support, resources and sense of belonging from these groups positively contribute to your overall wellbeing, mental health and job satisfaction.

**Making a difference:** Through advocating for diversity, equity and inclusion, these groups drive positive changes in policies, practices and culture, creating a more inclusive and equitable workplace for all employees like you.

**Boosting engagement and morale:** Engaging with these groups increases your commitment to the organization, enhances morale and creates a more positive work environment that boosts productivity.

**Recognizing customer diversity:** As we navigate a diverse world, these groups can help your organization better understand and meet the needs of your diverse customer base, leading to improved customer relations and a competitive edge in the market.

A well-resourced employee support network can transform company culture from the inside out and create a workplace where people not only accept, but embrace and celebrate neurodiversity, helping not only neurodivergents but all employees feel valued, welcome and empowered to bring their authentic selves to work.

Following a diagnosis of ADHD in adulthood, you may find yourself questioning many aspects of your life – your work and career choices included. Does your working environment support you or place extra demands on you that make it more difficult for you to do your job? If the latter, what practical steps could you or your employer take to improve the situation? After all, if you are in a stronger position to shine at work, everybody stands to benefit.

Remember that advocating for yourself and looking for the support you need are important to your mental wellbeing and chances to succeed at work. By tapping in to the power of community, you can create a more supportive environment for not only yourself but other neurodivergents who also need support in your workplace, driving a cultural change.

# Step 8:
# Find Your Community

Pursuing a late ADHD or AuDHD diagnosis is a process that can bring about a tsunami of upheaval in our lives. As we've seen, it's a highly individual journey that can open us up to a whole new world of discovery about ourselves, leaving our lives forever changed. Along the way, there will be those stories you tell yourself, and those you share with the world. Loneliness and depression can ensue when there is a disconnection between the stories brewing inside yourself and what you're able to share with the people around you.

This is why finding a community who can connect with you at the exact point where you are, and go on that journey with you, can be like finally being able to breathe a sigh of relief. It's a validation of the most painful struggles you've endured and the answers you've been looking for, and it confirms there are other people out there who understand and who will be able to commiserate with you.

In Step 8 of the ADHD iceberg, we're going to look at what it means to gain membership of the neurodiverse community and to find a support network so you don't have to do life alone.

### FINDING THE TRAVEL COMPANIONS YOU NEED

I know from experience how the discovery of what constitutes my neurotype brought about a profound sense of disconnect from who I was and my old life – the one I led before I knew what I was made of. I realized that my traits went beyond masking and that I'd developed an entire 'false self' when I was a child as a parentified daughter who had to be the mediator for her parents in the midst of their heated arguments. Growing up, I had taken this childhood conditioning and this 'self' into every interaction and relationship I went on to have in adulthood. This version of me was so inauthentic that all the parts inside me went to war every time I was called to make a big decision in my life.

So, it's no surprise to me now that when I first started trauma therapy, I told my then-husband I wanted a divorce that very same week. Therein my 'life-quake' began, as I found myself facing the prospect of life as a co-parent with two children aged under nine while juggling a growing social impact company. Whichever way you look at it, it was a major life transition. I had ripped my internal and external lives apart in order to rebuild a new me. I had to hit pause on my plans, go inward, and deal with all the pain that was brewing within.

I sought various means to release my trauma – through therapy, Pilates, yoga, mantra meditation, spiritual practices, my life purpose – and I sat with the pain. Importantly, I connected with people who were on the same journey and I took solace from those who had been where I was and who had emerged happier.

## HEADING WHERE YOU WANT TO GO

On your own journey, you'll likely grow tired of the recurring patterns in your relationships. And if you don't see them, the people around you will. The challenges that surface in our relationships can hold up a mirror in which we can truly see for the first time how we are showing up. Your partner or confidante may or may not have the psychological tools to help you unpack this, and you may eventually have to find your own way. That's when it can be especially comforting to realize that although you might have to do this by yourself, you aren't on your own, but part of a wider community.

As a collective, many of us are beginning to rebel against inauthenticity, or rather, against the need to fit in as anything other than ourselves. In our quest to find out who we are, we question our place in the world and we may feel adrift in a sea of people we'd known forever. But are we really alone? True empowerment begins when we know we can stand alone, and yet rely on others.

When so many of us are grappling with how to move forward following a life-changing diagnosis, there has never been a more important time to be a part of something bigger than us as an antidote to loneliness, depression and isolation. Lots of us may take the medication but we're allergic to being talked down to by healthcare professionals and are drawn to the empowering lived-experience narratives shared within the neurodiverse community. We long for a new tribe that understands what it is like to walk in these shoes, a community that validates our struggles; to walk together, and to compare notes at a time when we distrust a system that is supposedly made to treat and support us, but often seems to strip the power from us to run our lives.

**Reflection**
What strengths could you derive from being a part of a support network that truly understands your needs?

## THE POWER OF COMMUNITY

If most of us can agree on one thing, it's that life is easier when we have a support network in which we have each other's backs – where we provide support to each other, knowing it is reciprocated too.

To find out more about the power of community, I ran a poll in 2024 with my LinkedIn community, asking, 'What does community mean to you?' Of the respondents, 74 per cent said that they were looking for a place to belong and connect with like-minded people, 12 per cent said it's a place where they can be validated for who they are, and 11 per cent saw it as a place to look for support among people who understand. Recurring themes included:

**Solidarity:** a place that provides a sense of belonging and connection based on shared experience.

**Acceptance and mutual support:** being a part of a like-minded and compassionate community that promotes a sense of self-discovery, helps us feel seen and understood for who we are, and encourages us to express our beliefs and values.

**Representation matters:** it matters who you learn about neurodivergence and mental health matters from. Learning from the lived experience of those who foster an understanding of the specific challenges and joys experienced by different identities can help us to develop a more positive sense of identity and sharpen our self-perception and acceptance.

**Sharing contexts:** sharing lived experiences with a group of people from similar life contexts allows us to compare notes and provide support through offering relevant perspectives.

**Common interests:** facilitating connection through conversations, habits and routines built on common interests and hobbies.

**Trust built from altruism:** giving without expecting anything in return is seen as a positive and healing practice that can lead to personal growth and strengthening relationships through having each other's backs, which builds trust.

**Accessibility:** a community that can be accessed from our safe spaces and also provides in-person check-ins when our mental states change.

When we strip it all back, a community really boils down to one thing: that someone, somewhere understands what it feels like to be us. Through sharing experiences and support, we are participating in an exchange of energy that enriches our lives. A compassionate community reminds us that we are interconnected and that we each have the power to help shape a more compassionate and caring society as a whole.

More than this, perhaps what we're all looking for is the power to run our own lives. In 2023, the World Health Organization (WHO) and United Nations (UN) explained how its approach to mental health would be centred on a whole person approach, told via lived experience, and on community support, stating that through community inclusion, individuals who experience mental health challenges 'can access equal opportunities and access to services and support to enable participation in all areas of life'.

As Bessel van der Kolk argues in *The Body Keeps the Score*,[1] the field of psychiatry takes the power away from the individual – and the power in terms of support and treatment is very much placed in the hands of 'experts' and 'specialists'. A community represents a more humane approach, respecting personal autonomy and independence, and responding to our immediate and longer-term needs, which are shaped by the social aspects and various forms of intersecting oppressions in our life in motion. A well-run community puts the decision-making back into the hands of the individual as a human being, not as a 'patient'.

## WHAT FILLS YOUR CUP?

As we know, not all neurodivergents are the same and each of us will have different capacities for social interactions. Some of us enjoy group interactions, whereas some will find this exhausting and much prefer one-to-one conversations. Some of us may like to lead, while others just want to take part and bask in the community vibe, or play a more passive role in it. But at the end of the day, we are all seeking a sense of connection so we feel less alone and more supported.

As there are rich nuances in our neurodiverse experiences that are shaped by our diverse backgrounds, the things we need support for and the strategies that will actually work for us will differ from person to person, and from moment to moment. Remember that even if we share some of the same traits as another neurodivergent person, there will always be nuances caused by our diverse circumstances.

I'm still exploring the validity of trying to medicate away or extinguish some of the most widely publicized neurodivergent traits, as whether these traits become expressed as strengths or challenges depends a lot on our individual circumstances. For example, many of the ADHD traits that might be problematic in a structured environment which favours adherence to rules – for example impulsivity, distractibility or reward-seeking behaviours – can be an advantage in entrepreneurship, where exploratory and sensation-seeking traits can lead to the discovery of new avenues that no one has yet discovered.

Similarly, potential AuDHD challenges in maintaining eye contact, which can create difficulties in social interactions, aren't a problem in an environment where people understand that having eye contact can be very uncomfortable and may even elicit a fear response in these individuals. Moreover, many autistic individuals excel in the fields of science, technology, engineering and mathematics, which require deep solitary focus and study, and where relatively little eye contact is necessary anyway, only brain power.

Let's not forget that many of the challenges neurodivergents face can be similar to those experienced by individuals who face poverty, gender or racial biases and who can have feelings of isolation and discrimination that stem from living in a society that is made for a dominant culture that marginalizes them. In our isolation, joys and discoveries, there are parallels in our journey born from the experience of just being human.

## HEALING TOGETHER

An empowered community not only provides validation and a place to belong, but also facilitates recovery from mental health challenges among its members. The WHO and UN guide on mental health rights states that:

> 'The meaning of recovery can be different for each person and may include (re)gaining meaning and purpose in life; being empowered and able to live a self-directed life; strengthening the sense of self and self-worth; having hope for the future; healing from trauma; and living a life with purpose. Every person should have the opportunity to define what recovery means for them, and which areas of their life they wish to focus on as part of their

own recovery journey. Recovery considers the person and their context as a whole, and no longer adheres to the idea or goal of the person "being cured" or "no longer having symptoms."[2]

Recovery essentially means that we regain or stay in control of our lives, and being part of a community can help us in this respect.

When we go through conflicts in our lives in isolation, negative thought patterns can ensue and we may find ourselves catastrophizing about situations that aren't nearly as dire as we think. This is when it can be helpful to be part of a community that can give us a sense of perspective.

I've seen whole rooms light up from listening to someone share their stories and more importantly, the mindset and action that help facilitate their way of moving forward, their recovery from a lifetime of being confused about the ways their brain works. Similarly, at many of the public talks I've given, audience members have told me afterwards that they recognized a part of themselves in the stories I and others shared, which made them feel that they weren't alone, changed their perception about themselves, and gave them the courage to believe that they had everything and more within them to move forward and be a part of the change themselves.

## What Type of Community Works for You?

So, what community suits you? Here are some key areas you may wish to consider when looking for connection. Take a moment to reflect on these now and jot down your thoughts in response to the prompts:

1. **What does community mean for you?** Perhaps a support network to call upon when you are stuck, someone who understands, to feel more connected and less alone, or tips and strategies to navigate study, work and life.

> 2. **What type of community helps you feel you belong?** Perhaps one specific to your gender, culture, race, religious beliefs, life stages (such as being the working parent of neurodivergent children), relationships, divorce, single parenting, street community or shared interests and hobbies.
> 3. **What support are you looking for?** Emotional, mental, companionship, practical support in your career, business or childcare.
> 4. **Are you looking for one-to-one connection or a group to belong to and do activities together?**
> 5. **What are your interests and preferred activities?** Perhaps wellness, travelling, nature adventures, theatre, acting or art.
> 6. **How often do you want to participate in this community?** Weekly, monthly or ad hoc.
>
> Now that you've identified your unique needs, where do you go next?

## HOW TO FIND YOUR COMMUNITY

There are so many communities out there which provide support, resources and a sense of belonging. Many of them operate virtually, while some offer in-person meet-ups through events that bring the community together.

Depending on your life stage, you may be looking for a community to support you in navigating not only your neurodivergence but also your unique life situation through spending time with people who have similar interests or responsibilities to you.

Which path could you take to look for a community that caters to your current needs?

Talking to other adults with similar experiences who are committed to finding themselves and helping each other can be a positive experience which will help you with grounding your emotions, offer understanding, resources, a connection and a sense of belonging.

## Practical Ways to Find Your People

Review your replies to the exercise 'What Type of Community Works for You?' on page 255. Keeping those answers in mind, use the following toolkit to help you look for a community, jotting down your answers:

1. **Identify what you need at this stage of your life**
   - What life stage are you at?
   - What are the biggest challenges that you are facing right now?
   - What support do you need?
2. **Think about what you want to get out of being part of a community**
   - Clearly state your goals for participating in a community to determine if you're in the right place and if your needs will be met.
   - Think about how often and when you need to access the community.
3. **Which leader of a community do you connect to and resonate with?**
   - Is there a community leader whose views, tones, ethics and values you appreciate?
4. **In what setting would you be comfortable participating in the community?**
   - Do you prefer a one-to-one or group interaction?
   - What is your sharing style? For example, do you prefer to sit back and observe others, or do you prefer to share your challenges openly?

5. **Identify the particular areas for which you are seeking support and connection**
    - Is it important for you to be a part of a community that represents your intersectional identity, for example neurodiverse, gender, race, religion, social class and so on?
    - Are you seeking companionship with people who want to pursue similar interests, activities and hobbies?
    - Are you looking for support for your current life stage, for example as a carer, parenting, post-divorce or relationships?
6. **Research the community you are looking for**
    - Research online. Look for communities and forums for neurodivergents. Many charities and social impact companies such as ADHD UK, ADHD Foundation, ADHD Girls, Autistic Girls, Autism Women and Non-binary Network offer group support, drop-in sessions, and virtual and live events that enable people to connect, learn and support each other. Seek out neurodiversity-affirming groups on social media that you resonate with.
    - Look for local support groups. Try to find any neurodivergence charities, mental health support groups or local meet-up groups.
    - Workplace support groups. Check with HR if your employer has an employee resource group (ERG) set up to support their neurodivergent employees. Organizations like ADHD Girls, Institute of Neurodiversity, Neurodiversity in Business and Future is ND host online and in-person workshops, conferences and events for neurodivergents, employees and employers.
7. **Research grants and funding to access the support you need**
    For example, Access to Work in the UK offers grants up to £69,260 per year per individual and includes a provision for a mental health community or support workers via coaching and mentoring.[3]

## THE KEY TO RESPECTFUL COMMUNICATION

Remember that even if we are united by neurodivergence, each person's experience is unique, so it's important to approach any interactions with respect and empathy.

Within the neurodiverse community, there is such a rich diversity of experiences, which are not only shaped by our different overlapping identities but also by our different life stages. Even though we are united by the journey we are on, we are all at different stages, seasons and evolution within it, going through different levels of unravelling and reconciling with who we are. Because of your evolving understanding about your own neurodivergence, the conversations that you have with others will also likely refresh as you go, and you may discover that while there are some connections and opinions that you will resonate with, there will be others that you may struggle to see eye to eye with.

So how do you strike up conversations on these matters? Below, you will find some prompts to help you to self-advocate with your education settings, workplace and closest relationships.

1. **Evaluate the environment or person you want to open up to about your label to suss out their:**

   - Awareness levels
   - Cultural and familial beliefs about the label
   - Relationship quality with you
   - Likelihood of understanding

2. **If you're sure you want to open up about your neurodivergence, this is how you can talk about yourself:**

   - **Reframe neurodivergence as natural diversity:** explain that your neurodivergence is a brain difference that is as natural as biodiversity; it's just that the world hasn't caught up yet with what this means – that around 15–20 per cent of the world's population are neurodiverse!
   - **Embrace positive language, even if it may seem unnatural at first:** reframe your neurodivergence and mental health

challenges from the perspective of your innate strengths and abilities, and explain how you may require some support to express your skills fully – this is the same for everyone to a degree, but you've been able to identify a few areas in particular that you need support for.

- **Outline both your internal and external challenges:** the things you need support for aren't just based on your executive functioning, emotional regulation and other neurodivergent traits, but also on how well you are able to thrive within the daily reality of your circumstances. If you have invisible challenges, you may struggle even when given what appear to be equal opportunities as others within the same environment.
- **Ask for adjustments and discuss strategies that work for you as an individual:** what you need will be different to what another person needs, and will vary; for example, you may need cognitive, mental health, lifestyle or practical support in maintaining your household, emotional connections, communications and more.
- **Emphasize the importance of acceptance, understanding and autonomy:** it's important to reiterate that when we are in an environment that understands and accepts us for who we are, supports us without infantilizing or micromanaging us, and allows us to be autonomous, there's no telling how far we can go alone and together.
- **State the possibility that your needs will evolve over time:** mention that you are still learning as you go, and that you would appreciate it if they can show some patience as you continue to learn more about yourself. Some people have found themselves in the position of being infantilized or micromanaged and this isn't what you want.
- **Remark on the collective attitudes outside your setting:** state that the paradigm is shifting towards neurodiversity being viewed as a completely natural way of being and that many neurodiversity advocates, including high-profile celebrities, are working towards changing society's perception and busting the stigma.

3. **Maintain an open mind in your communication**

- Seek to understand other people's perspectives before you speak up.
- Use assistive technologies to help you transcribe verbal conversations into written scripts so you can review conversations and take note of what you missed.
- Understand that it may occasionally take you a little time to process a conversation, so you may need a follow-up conversation.
- Accept what neurodivergence means to each person and that we all have different views. Try to adopt a balanced view, in which everyone is approaching the issue from the perspective of their own individual experiences.

## LEARNING AS WE GO

I'm certainly not saying that I've always got communication right. I'm still often susceptible to an all-or-nothing mentality. For example, once on a financial company's intersectionality panel, I said that it was easier to advocate for yourself the longer you've worked within a company – to the dismay of someone who observed that it didn't matter how long you worked in a company, it still might not be easy if the culture wasn't inclusive.

When I first founded ADHD Girls, I received many messages from neurodivergent men, trans, non-binary and other identities asking for a place in my community. At times when I've posted about the realities of neurodivergent women on LinkedIn, I get a kickback from neurodivergent men who feel underrepresented and say they wish I'd created ADHD Men instead, because they too need tangible support.

On the surface, neurodivergent men may pass as the dominant culture that society was built for. However, because they've had to mask their differences while flying under the radar, this has caused them significant challenges from the expectations placed on them, too. I'm sure that for every man who's contributed to the statistics of mental health challenges, more have hidden in plain sight because of the struggle to show their vulnerability or the lack of a place for them to do so. I think this shows that we shouldn't leave anyone behind, and real meaningful social changes can only happen when we bring everyone along on the journey.

That said, for every man who thinks that I'm reinforcing stereotypes that frame masking or less obvious forms of neurodivergence as experiences that are exclusive to women and girls and that due to the dominant culture, men are able to mask easier, I think we're missing the point here. True belonging is about seeing the big picture of our collective experiences, and still opening up about the challenges we face if we belong to an underrepresented group. It's okay to highlight the plight of those who perhaps feel they don't have a voice and bring this to the fore. We need to emphasize the diversity of experiences, which isn't about perpetuating stereotypes, but brings more awareness to our collective consciousness.

There was a time very early on in my career advocating for those with ADHD when I realized in the middle of the night that I haven't written a social media post, so I quickly wrote one with a blasé hook: 'Is ADHD a disability? Let's change that shall we?' – and found I'd been trolled up to my eyeballs when I woke up the next day. There will be those whose ADHD has landed them in the scrapheap of life and they are really disabled by the condition. And yes, I know this. What appeared frivolous to others came from my own experience of having found myself in murky waters as an AuDHDer who was trying to choose the healthier way of life, rather than one who was still caught up in self-medicating and repeated cycles of destruction that were harmful to myself and those around me. But to others, my post would have seemed inconsiderate and insensitive, I appreciate that.

These are all clumsy encounters that I often share with my friend Joseph Pack, the founder of Drug Free ADHD, who has had his fair share of disgruntled neurodivergent members of the public criticizing his social media posts. Rather than inducing a state of polarization within those who identify with the traits within the same label, let's remember that we are all still learning. As you and the world catch up with what it means to be a neurodivergent and our individual ways of moving forward, let's just assume that we don't know anything yet and that we can keep learning from one another. I find that it's when people say I'm wrong that I learn. So please be open to learning about the collective neurodiverse experience, especially if you want to be part of the social change.

## MOBILIZING SOCIAL CHANGE

Within the neurodiverse community, we all have our favourite lived experience advocates who uncover hidden stories from so many parts of our lives. When a neurodivergent from an underrepresented group speaks up about the issues that they face, they plant seeds of change that bring clarity to conditions that have so far been under-researched and poorly represented, particularly for people with marginalized identities.

For so many late-diagnosed neurodivergents, the realization later in life that we have been missed sparks a mission to help others. Many of us attempt to heal our pain through a process of, for example:

- Absorbing every podcast, article, book and YouTube video about the topic.
- Setting up our own podcasts to speak to other neurodivergent people or experts to gain a deeper understanding and some free advice.
- Harbouring a deep yearning to create a platform, group, community or other entity that not only creates a way for like-minded people to come together, but also acts as a force for change.

Creating change takes strength, determination and boots on the ground. This is especially true in those situations where we feel outnumbered, alone and isolated, because there is strength in numbers. I often get approached by neurodivergents who work in companies that have yet to hold any neurodiversity awareness sessions or create a neurodiversity employee resource group. The prospect of opening up to others about their diagnosis can then become incredibly scary as the first person to take on an entire establishment, in the face of an unpredictable response to their diagnosis and the potential stigma. There is a fear of being misunderstood and judged for something that is so inherent in their way of being, as well as the fear of losing their job. It can feel incredibly lonely – but we are not alone.

During the hardest times of our lives, when challenges with our interactions and relationships can trigger our trauma wounds, it's important to hold sight of our experiences as being shared by the collective in certain respects. To banish the stigma from society, we first have to work on ourselves and replace any faulty beliefs that we're not good enough with self-acceptance and confidence so that we can begin to build a constructive path for ourselves and others.

## BECOME PART OF THE CHANGE YOU WANT TO SEE

If I had a penny for every time I'm asked, 'What can I do if I want to make a change?', I would be rich by now. But change is easier to enact than you think. I am a firm believer that by improving the lives of others, we can also facilitate healing within ourselves.

For every person who has asked me what they can do to drive the winds of change, I would say you can start by defining the following:

**Your mission:** understand the goal you are working towards.
**Your sphere of influence:** where is the immediate environment where you can promote solidarity and support?
**Who do you want to help:** children, adults or specific identities that you represent?
**Your interests and skills:** what are the skills you possess that you can channel towards creating an entity to be a part of the change? You could be a media campaigner, author, speaker, coach, counsellor,

therapist, entrepreneur, wellness practitioner, charity volunteer, policy campaigner or something else.

**Time and money:** can you spare time, attention and money on your mission, as it's very likely you will be working for no money for a time?

**How you will balance spending time on your purpose with self-care:** you are neurodivergent after all, with very real physical, mental, emotional and social-health needs.

### Where Do Neurodivergents Need Support?

If you need any inspiration for areas that neurodivergents need support within different sections of society, here are the places you could start exploring:

- Health policy and funding for services and assessments to help more people access diagnosis and support.
- Campaigning for better public understanding that neurodiversity is to be embraced as diversity of the human mind, not a condition that is somehow 'less than'.
- Training of healthcare professionals around neurodivergence that takes a person-centred, intersectional and holistic approach.
- Working within neurodivergent healthcare and support services.
- Research and development of rating and masking scales that can be used by underrepresented groups.
- Women's health research, such as the impact of hormones on neurodivergent women.
- Creating positive groups that inspire and support neurodivergents in school, college and university, with emphasis on supporting their transitionary stages.
- Community groups for neurodivergents.

- Neurodiversity advocate and speaker aiming to promote neurodiversity awareness through an intersectional and trauma-informed lens within schools, community groups and organizations.
- Creating an employee resource group within your organization and encouraging people to come together.
- Practical and wellbeing support for neurodivergents across their major life transitions, such as puberty, marriage, parenthood, pregnancy, childbirth, menopause, divorce, grief and bereavement, sickness, rehab, accidents, caring responsibilities, discrimination incidences and other stressful life situations.

## WHY DO YOU WANT CHANGE?

I think we need to truly align with the reasons *why* we want to make a change. Personally, I wanted to set up a platform to amplify the voices of neurodivergent women from all backgrounds and enable them to share how ADHD presents for them. Enabling us to express ourselves marks the start of increasing our representation. And when I started talking about the experiences of neurodivergent women and girls, this opened up doors for me to speak about the experiences of intersectional identities, like mine, which helps shape the ways in which neurodiversity manifests in our lives. When this issue is featured on social media, this then allows many others to feel seen and validated, and sparks healing within themselves. It hands the power back to the individual and helps them regain a sense of autonomy in their lives.

By working in neurodiversity and intersectionality and dissecting how the multiple degrees of overlap contribute to the outcome of privilege or oppression, I have been able to see the parallels in our stories. There is a connection in our human experiences that reflects our shared humanity – that we are all in so many ways alike when we encounter joys and challenges as a result of our unique biology and life circumstances. We don't need to be neurodivergent to face disablement, for example, as if we were unfortunate to suffer from illness or get into an accident at any stage in our lives, we would still be disabled by society.

Similarly, the life stage of menopause is a commonality among women, so neurodivergent or not, if we are biologically female, we will in all likelihood face varying degrees of challenges at some point during this pivotal time of our lives. It is important to emphasize, though, that depending on many interacting factors such as biological differences, access to good-quality healthcare, and the quality of our significant relationships, a neurodivergent woman may or may not find her challenges compounded during menopause.

Ultimately, if we can bridge the empathy gap between the neuro-labelled and neuro-not-yet-labelled through understanding the nuances of our experiences, which have so far been simplified, we will be able to build a new society that blurs the lines between labels and creates a sense of unity, safety, belonging and meaningful support for all. We will be working towards creating a society that is built for diverse ways of being. We each have a way of affecting each other, for better or worse. In my book, it's always worth bringing a balanced perspective to spark positive actions to create a sense of belonging for those who, for so long, have felt marginalized and excluded in society.

Every neurodivergent activist who sets out to mobilize social change will experience considerable pushback along the way. The journey can be likened to pushing a boulder up a hill, where you will find yourself refining your stance as you state your case for change. The irony is that the process of elevating the rights of an underrepresented group can at times make you feel disconnected from the community you live in. You are creating a new society, after all.

For each person who wants to make a significant social change, there is another who wants to make a difference on a smaller scale. This work may begin outwardly, but along the way, you will very likely come to realize that the focus and fervour with which you pour your attention and love into the world will eventually shine an overwhelmingly bright light back onto you. Along the way, you may also stop and start, get burned out, isolate yourself from those closest to you as you obsess about your mission, and you will question why you sometimes spend more time on your purpose than those who need you. This is when you will be challenged to go inward and strengthen the muscles you've built to stand strong and tall.

This journey will ultimately walk you home to yourself, and help you see that every intention you set out to change the world for the better can be a reflection of the parts of you that are still looking for answers, which have yet to be revealed – the parts that are seeking love and belonging in your new day-to-day reality.

The route ahead is open to you to make what you want from it. When you seek to belong in a community, you may at times encounter a tension between your need for connection and acceptance, and your personal authenticity that has always been there from your childhood. Belonging isn't just about finding a group or community – it's about finding a community where you don't have to sacrifice your authenticity in order to belong, and which honours and respects your true self. Finding that balance can be difficult, especially when group dynamics challenge your individuality. Emotional maturity and self-awareness often come from learning how to handle these tensions with resilience – ultimately finding spaces (both internal and external) where you can be your true self and still belong.

At a time when so many of us are turning inward and becoming increasingly more self-centred, there is something to be said about reflecting on what is most important to us at this stage of our lives.

This is when you search within and ask yourself what you value and what life you want for yourself. For example, are you the sort of person who values vocation, purpose and meaning, or do you value the comforts of belonging? Because I've found it incredibly hard to reconcile my own need for authenticity and my need for attachment, having been tested time and time again on this. And I still don't have all the answers. I just know that my wild heart needs to choose my mission and that I must then breathe life fully into it as I've done in the past.

# Step 9:
# Emerge as Your True Self

Congratulations, you made it here! Together, we've excavated into the layers beneath the tip of the ADHD iceberg and now it's time to come up for air. Receiving an ADHD diagnosis later in life, or coming to terms with the fact that you may need one, can feel like someone finally handed you a map – only to realize it's written in a language that doesn't quite capture the journey you've travelled.

Many of us come to this diagnosis not as a clean slate but as people who have already survived so much: misdiagnosis, masking, misunderstanding, trauma, cultural conditioning and often co-occurring conditions like anxiety, depression, chronic pain and undiagnosed autism.

And here's the kicker: until 2013, psychiatry didn't officially recognize that ADHD and autism could co-occur. With the DSM-5 (*Diagnostic and Statistical Manual of Mental Disorders*) came a loosening of rigid diagnostic boundaries – and with it, an acknowledgement of what so many of us have known all along: that human neurodiversity doesn't slot neatly into categories. That many of us are not 'just ADHD' or 'just autistic', but complex and intersecting; for example, we might be AuDHDers with PTSD and potentially other 'D's, with layers that reflect our lived realities far more than any symptom checklist ever could.

Healthcare professionals, under increasing pressure to make sense of rising diagnoses, are now tasked with the impossible: trying to decode our internal worlds from the outside. But as we explored in Step 1, how can they fully grasp what we've lived through if they haven't lived it themselves? If they don't understand the identities we've shaped – as a result of factors like gender, culture, race, class, queerness, trauma and the long years of not knowing why we were different – how can they truly interpret the ways we cope, collapse or cry for help?

ADHD treatment still largely focuses on increasing neurotransmitters, cognitive strategies and psychoeducation. And while those things can help, they're only a small part of the picture. Are our educational models keeping up with what we now know? Or are we simply repackaging the same ideas for a population that looks and lives very differently?

The *New York Times* article 'Have We Been Thinking About ADHD All Wrong?' highlights just how complex this picture has become.[1] Decades of research still haven't identified a clear biological marker for ADHD. Many people experience symptoms that fluctuate over time, disappear or re-emerge depending on their life circumstances. ADHD, the author surmised, may not be a fixed, lifelong disorder in the way we once thought – but a context-sensitive condition, heavily influenced by environment, trauma and identity.

Medications like Ritalin and Adderall can improve focus or behaviour in the short term, but research shows these effects often fade – and they don't necessarily improve academic performance or life satisfaction. What they *do* reliably change is emotion: making tasks feel more engaging, but not necessarily making us more effective.

And here's what might be the most ground-breaking shift: many researchers now suggest that ADHD is not a black-and-white diagnosis, but a continuum – a spectrum of traits, shaped by both biology and life circumstance. The more we learn, the more we see that ADHD is not just about what's inside your brain – it's about how your brain interacts with the world around you.

So, what does this mean for us, in real time? It means that no one-size-fits-all strategy will ever be enough. Every piece of advice we take on board and every choice we make – from the tools we use, to the rest we allow ourselves – needs to pass through the filter of who we are and what we've lived through. Our neurodivergence is not a fixed identity; it's a moving landscape, shaped by biology, relationships, trauma, transitions and culture. Let's explore what it means to live well with that kind of complexity.

In Step 9, I'm going to be offering you tools and strategies based on all we've discovered so far, which are designed to help you face the future empowered by self-awareness and self-belief. While there may be more surprises to come on the path ahead, remember that you are a member of the wider ADHD community, and as such, you're not in this alone.

## OUR LIVES IN MOTION

Understanding ADHD or AuDHD isn't just about traits – it's about learning to see the whole system you live inside. Our existential reality is multi-layered, with each layer adding depth to our humanity – the culmination of a dynamic interaction between our biology and everything we've been through in life, which affects our cognitive, mental, physical and emotional health. As multi-layered beings, we exist in a constant state of flux, in which our behaviour, ability to regulate our emotions, how we act in different situations, quality of our relationships and ability to handle life's challenges will all be subjected to many different factors.

To understand the ever-changing landscape of how your ADHD or AuDHD manifests in your life in motion and how to regain balance when you feel out of sync, you will need to become aware of the following interconnected systems.

### 1. Your current biological state

Your internal biology can have profound effects on your health and wellbeing, shaping your experiences, perspectives and interactions with the world. This can be reflected in your body's systems, as illustrated by some of the common challenges seen in ADHD and AuDHD.

**Nervous system:** executive function challenges, social anxiety, coordination challenges, hyperactivity, impulsivity, overactive thinking loop and big emotions

**Stress response system:** chronic stress, burnout, fight-or-flight response, overwhelm

**Gut and immune system:** nutrient deficiencies, blood sugar imbalances, leaky gut, gut dysbiosis

**Sensory system:** sensory integration differences

**Endocrine system:** hormonal fluctuations and detoxification

**Detoxification and inflammatory system:** heavy metal, catecholamine, toxin load

**Cardiovascular system:** heart arrythmia, low heart rate variability, high blood pressure

**Circadian system:** atypical sleep–wake cycle, sleep apnoea, restless leg syndrome, insomnia, delayed sleep phase syndrome, hormonal symptoms that interfere with sleep

These imbalances are not your fault. Many of them are invisible burdens you've been carrying silently for years. You are not broken – your system may simply be overwhelmed or out of sync with what you truly need.

## 2. Your surroundings and circumstances

How you perceive and experience physical spaces, social interactions, responsibilities, support or your level of freedom and security will greatly influence how you respond or react to your surroundings, and ultimately, how your neurodivergence is expressed. We may be especially sensitive to sounds, smells, sight, vibes and moods of people, places and things, and may try to find ways to cope with this and become very malleable to our surroundings over time.

## 3. Support network and relationships

Being understood, accepted and having supportive people around us, friends, family members and positive role models, can make a big difference in how we experience our neurodivergence. These supportive factors can give us strength and encouragement to face the challenges that come with our neurodivergent traits.

### 4. Opportunities and trauma

The experiences of opportunities and traumas we encounter in life play a significant role in influencing how we show up. Our responses and adaptations to these important life events, guided by societal influences and our personal circumstances, can shape our perceptions of success, failure and of our strengths, talents, confidence and worthiness. As trauma colours the lens through which we see the world, we may have default responses and communication patterns that can lead to misunderstandings in our interactions and relationships.

### 5. Life transitions and stages

For neurodivergent individuals, life transitions can be especially challenging – these are times when the demands of change and adaptation outweigh their capacity to cope, often leading to heightened stress and overwhelm. Demands can come from minor transitions or large life-changing events such as pregnancy, childbirth, menopause, marriage, parenthood, sickness, quitting an addiction to drugs and alcohol, rehab, accidents, bereavement, break up, divorce, transition to university, starting a new job, moving to a new place or experiencing significant life milestones. All these things impact our neurodiverse experiences.

### 6. Social and cultural influence

These are the pressures and expectations placed on us by the society, the norms and values of the culture we live in, and the duties we feel towards others. These factors can affect how we manage our neurodiverse experiences. The messages we continue to get from society and the beliefs instilled by our culture can shape how we view and react to our neurodivergence.

### 7. Nurture

Everything that happened from our time in the womb to our entry into the world, including our susceptibility to intergenerational trauma or support, the things that happened to us and within us as children growing up through puberty, adolescence, young adulthood, adulthood and the rest of our lives.

## 8. Nature

The genes we inherited from our parents, which can be passed along to our children. Our genetic story may reveal our propensity towards certain conditions and how our biology works. Our genes may also influence the choices we make to gravitate towards a certain outcome, which affects our health for better or for worse. However, the expression of our genes may be changed via epigenetics, depending on how we live our lives, the people we have around us, and whether we take care of our mental and physical wellbeing.

We need to consider the dynamic interplay of elements in our life in motion, so we can gain a deeper understanding of how our neurodivergence evolves at different stages of our life and influences our experiences as we navigate the complexities of the world around us. Underneath the challenges of emotional and physical dysregulation, there are layers of conditioning that at times make us forget that *there is a place that is always at rest within us*. A place that we can tap into, one which we were all born with. A place of peace that is ever elusive to those of us living a life in the fast lane. To be able to return to this place at any given moment, we need to create space to settle our minds – whether it's before or after our response to an emotional trigger. It is through this sort of reflection that we will unravel the hidden depths of our being, discovering reserves of resilience, wisdom and a profound connection to the vast complexities of our shared human experience.

### Reflection

Take a moment now to read through these interconnected systems again. Are you aware of any traits or patterns that suggest your current approach to living with ADHD or AuDHD might need some adjusting? What practical steps could help you realign and better support yourself, moving forward?

## HOW TO TUNE INTO YOURSELF AND KEEP YOUR SEPARATE PARTS IN HARMONY

In your personal excavation of the layers that comprise the ADHD iceberg, you might start noticing that things aren't as random or erratic as they've always seemed. That which may appear 'all over the place' from the outside – the swinging between go-with-the-flow chaos and iron-fisted control – is actually something much more nuanced: your nervous system trying to keep you afloat in a world that hasn't always met you with understanding.

Underneath it all, there might be something quieter – something closer to the truth of who you are: the Self, which isn't a single, unified entity, but rather an entire community of separate parts shaped by survival, longing and hope that show up to protect, perform or persevere in our relationships and day-to-day lives. When these parts reflect opposing drives, it can be incredibly exhausting, and often, it's our autonomic nervous system – not our conscious Self – that's steering the ship. This isn't a flaw, but a signal that something in you knows there's more truth, more vital life force within you that is waiting to surface and be heard.

To come home to yourself, you'll need to become fluent in the language of your inner world. This means tending to the exiled, forgotten and over-functioning parts of yourself with understanding and care. In this respect, I'm a fan of Richard Schwartz's Internal Family Systems (IFS) model[2] – not as a doctrine, but as a helpful lens. The IFS is an integrative approach to individual psychotherapy. Schwartz himself identifies as being an ADHDer, and developed IFS as a way of understanding that the mind naturally has 'parts' – or what other schools of thought might call sub-personalities, ego states or voices. Perhaps as a way to adapt to our upbringings and an ever-changing world of demands, we've developed some parts that might have served us well in the past, but which have now become a barrier to us having fulfilling relationships with ourselves and others. It's important to understand that these parts aren't necessarily the direct results of our ADHD or AuDHD, but that they are shaped by our experiences as a result of living with neurodivergence in the world.

The idea isn't to silence or override these parts; it's to get curious about them and build relationships with them. To hear what they are trying to say, because when we can lead ourselves from a place of awareness and compassion, rather than fear or reactivity, something shifts. IFS talks about the 8Cs of self-leadership: calmness, clarity, curiosity, compassion, confidence, courage, creativity and connectedness. You don't need to nail them all at once. Just notice where you already have access to them, and where you might need to make space. Where you're gripping too tight. Where you're holding your breath. Where you've been armouring up, when what you really need is softness and some anchors that you can return to as you begin to integrate the various different parts that comprise your unique identity (preferably with the support of a sympathetic therapist, if you can find one who gets it). They offer you a way to come back into alignment when everything feels out of sync.

## The Eight Cs of Self-leadership

If you were to work with a therapist, here's how you can apply a neurodivergent lens to IFS's 8Cs of self-leadership.

- **Calmness**

Our ability to tap into a state of calm can vary considerably, depending on our triggers. At lower levels of emotional intensity, we can employ soothing grounding methods such as practising mindfulness, meditation, yoga and breathwork, or playing with our pets. At a higher level of emotional distress, we may need to tap into tools to help soothe us in the immediate moment so we can respond in a reasonable way, rather than react in extreme and adverse ways to triggers. Tools we can use to manage moments of distress or overwhelm include splashing cold water on our face, biting into flavoured ice lollies, exiting the room and calming down in a dark room with dim lights or – at the other extreme – through engaging in intense exercise.

- Clarity

Differences in the ways in which we pay attention and process information, which can stem from the way in which we perceive everything at once, may cause us to view situations as being more severe than they really are. Our different parts may flare up all at once, but we can try to step outside them to observe them and understand their origins, and how they were shaped from our past experiences into the stories we tell ourselves about life.

- Curiosity

We have a natural desire to explore and understand more about a topic, event or person, which can help us evaluate how the life we have endured shows up in our current thoughts, emotions and ideas. As neurodivergents, we often have the ability to hold large chunks of information in our minds at the same time, so we need to recognize that mastering the different parts of ourselves isn't about diminishing one part and elevating another. Rather, it's about being aware of what they are, what they're showing us, and reframing the negative 'ending' associated with a traumatic memory, for example, and inviting the parts to enter into a more integrative state of peace.

- Compassion and Confidence

As our self-esteem may have suffered from a lifetime of being fed with negative messaging, we may need to outsource our confidence, at least at the start. For those who've had a particularly difficult start in life, your self-compassion may be close to non-existent and this is why you will need to be particularly aware of the language you use about yourself, refraining from judgement and viewing yourself with kindness instead. It is also worth recognizing how our parts may take on the burden of other people's suffering, especially of those we care for; some of our parts may in fact be carrying the projections of others onto us, rather than our own issues.

- **Courage and Creativity**

Many neurodivergents are naturally courageous and, as such, we need to accept responsibility for the role we play in situations. We also have an innate talent for creativity, able to produce original ideas in the face of an observation, and we should learn to trust in our capacity to handle life's challenges by creatively solving problems independently or collaboratively.

- **Connectedness**

We need to recognize that we are a part of a collective community of people sharing similar experiences, that we are connected to others and our actions have an impact on those in our immediate sphere and beyond. The beauty of this work lies in understanding how we bring ourselves into every interaction and relationship.

At its core, self-mastery isn't about control, it is about honouring the differences within us in order to create a coherent inner community. The more aware you are of your internal states and what you're made of, the more you'll be able to tap into inner wisdom and empathy, too. This will give you the tools to better regulate your emotions, and to master *you* – so you are better able to respond rather than react to others and change any unhelpful repeating patterns of behaviour.

## FINDING A STATE OF INNER CALM IN THE CHAOS

On my journey into learning how to regulate my own emotional triggers, I've discovered that regulation isn't about achieving permanent calm but about building capacity. The work is often about expanding the space between stimulus and response so I'm not constantly spiralling through the same reactive loops. To do that, I've had to widen my window of capacity (or window of tolerance) – the range in which I can stay present, grounded and connected to myself – and develop radical compassion towards those moments when I inevitably experience a shutdown or meltdown.

Touched upon earlier in Steps 5 and 6, the concept of the window of tolerance was originally developed by Dr Daniel Siegel, a renowned psychiatrist and neurologist, and represents the optimal state of arousal or stimulation in which we can function at our best and cope with stressors in a balanced manner. Within this window, we can think clearly, make decisions and learn efficiently, regulate our emotions, form positive and healthy relationships, and be flexible and adaptable. However, this state can be elusive in the world we find ourselves in. As neurodivergents who live with prolonged chronic stress, our nervous systems have a tendency to swing between opposite extremes – from a hyper-alert, overstimulated state into a hypo-arousal state, where we are numbed out and flattened.

Rather than trying to 'calm down' or 'be less reactive', I've found it more helpful to think in terms of integration. That means not just soothing the traits, but tuning in to the deeper, layered systems that make up who we are – body, brain, breath and relationship. When those systems are in connection with each other, we can move through the world in a more regulated, present and responsive way.

This kind of integration isn't about expecting ourselves to be perfect; for instance, being able to automatically lower the lever when we are in a hyper-stimulated state or to raise the lever when we are in hyper-arousal state. If you are looking for quick ways to shift your state, though, I've found that breathwork (for example, deep belly, longer exhale, box breathing), somatic movement (such as shaking out tension in my limbs, dancing and grounding my feet into the earth), as well as sitting in the bath are practices that speak directly to my nervous system in a language it understands. These practices say: you are safe now.

In his book *IntraConnected*,[3] Siegel identifies nine domains of integration. While there isn't space to go into his theory in detail here, what I love about this concept is that it offers a holistic view that marries the mind, body and relational aspects. Adapted for our purposes as ADHDers, the key takeaways include the following ideas.

### 1. An invitation to be aware of what is happening in our internal world

As neurodivergents, we often feel the world first before we know how to make sense of those sensory inputs. This is a call to cultivate mindfulness and compassion by connecting with our whole body. Slowing down to notice where tension or emotion sits in the body and giving it breath, movement or sound can help us metabolize whatever blockages we are holding and release them.

### 2. Encourage awareness of self-regulation

For ADHDers and AuDHDers, self-regulation can be a major challenge due to difficulties with social communication, sensory processing and emotional regulation. Overwhelming sensory input, both external and social, can interfere with processing information and lead to behaviours like stimming, which are actually self-soothing strategies. Avoiding social interactions can hinder the development of social skills, making it harder to engage in competent social communication. By integrating and harmonizing our internal parts, we can support better social interactions and move towards a healthier state over time.

### 3. Make the implicit explicit

Our actions as neurodivergents are driven by our conscious parts (what we see, hear and feel tangibly) and our unconscious agendas, desires and motivations. Giving voice to those parts – through journaling, creative expression, talking to a trusted friend or therapist – helps turn what's been unconscious into something we can finally understand and work with.

### 4. A shift to systems thinking

We are human beings whose bodies' interconnected systems work together in ways that impact how we show up. Simultaneously, our external world also impacts our internal world. It isn't a single cause and effect; for example, any emotional dysregulation we experience isn't solely due to a difference in our brains. Rather, our emotional dysregulation could be a result of multiple factors, such as biological pathways working together to affect different body systems, hormonal transitions, or responding to a throwaway comment that hits an old wound or a lifetime of coded expectations. When we stop blaming ourselves and start mapping the systems at play, we build understanding instead of shame.

5. **Interconnected relational aspects that transcend communities, cultures and beliefs**

An emphasis on the importance of interconnectedness and relational aspects of our being through honouring differences between our self and different relationships, and promoting linkages with others in the world.

Inner calm is a capacity we grow by returning to ourselves again and again, through the body, through the breath, through connection. You don't need to be perfect. You just need enough space – inside and around you – to move differently when life gets loud.

## The Wheel of Awareness Meditation

Siegel has created the Wheel of Awareness meditation, which can serve as a valuable tool for neurodivergent individuals to enhance their focus, expand their awareness, and cultivate kindness in their intentions.[4] The Wheel is a metaphor or a visual representation of how the mind works, sending our awareness to the first five senses, bodily sensations, mental activities and interconnection.

I've been doing this meditation daily and the benefits I've derived from it are:

- Changing my stressed state into one of balance of equanimity
- Balancing the two branches of my autonomic nervous system, the parasympathetic and sympathetic
- Lowering stress
- Helping unblock pressure in my heart centre and steadying my heart rate
- Tapping into that ever-elusive internal contentment on demand

## HOW TO KEEP 'YOU' AT THE CENTRE

How do you begin to devise a personalized approach to cater for a label like ADHD, which encompasses such a vast diversity of neurodiverse experiences? You need to tune in to what your personal challenges and protective factors are in your current life stage and circumstances.

As described in 'Mental Health, Human Rights and Legislation: Guidance and Practice' issued jointly by the World Health Organization (WHO) and Office of the United Nations High Commissioner for Human Rights (OHCHR), 'Recovery [from mental health challenges] is a personal process, different for every individual, and tied to self-determination, healing relationships, and social inclusion.'[5] A personalized approach to your label should therefore focus on understanding and respecting your individual differences and preferences to promote growth, autonomy and fulfilment. The following table offers some elements to consider.

By considering the elements in the table and centring your authentic needs in your life while honouring a sense of interdependence, you will not only enhance your quality of life and express yourself, but also foster a true sense of belonging through being mindful of your place in the collective. Honouring yourself as you move forward with your label will require a balance between being aware of your authentic needs within your internal world and understanding how your external world affects you.

| ELEMENT TO CONSIDER | AREA OF FOCUS |
|---|---|
| Your individual needs and preferences tailored to life stage, circumstances and context | **Life contexts:** what is currently a challenge that you need support to navigate? Are you aware of anything at your stage of life that may affect your neurodivergence, for example, lifestyle, stress, hormones, demands or medication?<br>**Physical, mental, emotional and sensory needs:** understanding how your biology and physiology determine your behaviours to tailor strategies that work better for you, for example medication, nutritional supplements, gut healing, lifestyle advice to regulate your neurotransmitter and stress levels, managing your energy, addiction recovery and supporting your health.<br>**Learning and processing:** awareness of your learning styles, whether this is primarily visual, auditory, kinaesthetic or a combination of these, in order to optimize learning outcomes and processing differences.<br>**Social-communication:** understanding your unique need for social connection which may differ to others, strengthening your capacities for developing social skills, and seeking support in understanding social cues to navigate social interactions. |
| Strengths-based approach | **Personal:** what strengths do you bring to every interaction? These could include being calm and able to think clearly under pressure, intelligence and creativity with problem-solving, empathy, compassion, creating routines and planning to give structure to your day, or skills to scan the future and anticipate challenges. |

*(Continued)*

| ELEMENT TO CONSIDER | AREA OF FOCUS |
|---|---|
| | **Education and career:** awareness and understanding of your unique talents, strengths and interests – and channelling this into doing something that the world needs and would pay for. Develop your own 'owner's manual' for when you can be most productive, adopt the tools you need to assist your learning and processing differences, seek neurodivergent career or work coaching or invest in personal and professional development. |
| Emotional regulation strategies to navigate daily interactions | **Tap into tools based on levels of emotional intensity:**<br>• Level 1: Mindfulness strategies (for example three deep belly breaths, body scan, noticing five things you can see/hear/feel).<br>• Level 2: Regulating emotions (for example gentle movement such as walking or stretching, journaling, naming the emotion out loud).<br>• Level 3: Distress tolerance (for example splashing cold water on your face, biting into a lemon or ice lolly, holding an ice cube, stepping into a dark or quiet space).<br>**Be mindful of the reasons that underlie your traits:** repeating patterns of behaviour may have links to traumatic imprints (hyper-arousal), sensory sensitivities, psychosocial stress (RSD) or biological stress (hormonal transitions), empathy gap, communication differences or absence of a support network. |

| ELEMENT TO CONSIDER | AREA OF FOCUS |
| --- | --- |
|  | **Long-term strategies to build emotional resilience:** try different therapeutic modalities that work for YOU to improve your reaction to emotional triggers; decide if medication is for you; consider practising mindfulness, meditation, spirituality or physical exercise; and nurture a support network of like-minded people who understand and give you a sense of belonging. |
| Communication skills to nurture your relationships | **Daily interactions:** adjust how you communicate to fit what works best for each person – whether they prefer talking, seeing, reading or other ways of connecting.<br>**Significant relationships:** visualize the ideal mood, emotions and thoughts you want to have in your significant relationships, to associate positive feelings with your interactions; model the culture you want to experience in your relationships; identify communication patterns that may harm relationships; increase awareness of triggers and reactions; practise active listening; express feelings openly and lovingly without blame; establish boundaries around communication; cultivate empathy and understanding towards your relationship partner; resolve conflict through using 'fair fighting' techniques, compromise and negotiation; and seek support and guidance from a therapist or counsellor to improve communication skills and address underlying issues in the relationship and break the cycle of intergenerational trauma. |

*(Continued)*

| ELEMENT TO CONSIDER | AREA OF FOCUS |
|---|---|
| Adjustments, collaborations and feedback | **Seek accommodation and adjustments in your environments:** this can be in your personal, study or work life to support your specific needs and enable you to bring your strengths to the situation and set you up for success.<br>**Collaboration and feedback:** involve another person in your environment to co-create strategies and solutions to make decisions that work for you both moving forward; be open to feedback to see if the approaches are effective and keep an open channel to improve. |
| Interdependence | **Fostering interdependence while also being authentic:** be open to the idea that you live in a relational context and that we are all affecting each other for better or for worse. Promote interdependence to foster abundance via:<br>• Fostering a culture centred on honest and transparent communication where everyone feels comfortable to express their true selves without fear of judgement.<br>• Providing mutual support and encouraging each other to help one another based on strengths and needs.<br>• Respecting individual differences.<br>• Promoting collaborative partnerships, and offering personalized support.<br>• Empowering each other to advocate for themselves and express needs and preferences assertively.<br>• Creating a safe and inclusive culture where everyone feels accepted, valued and respected.<br>• Fostering a culture of empathy, compassion and understanding to promote interdependence while honouring authenticity. |

As the Greek philosopher Aristotle said, 'The whole is greater than the sum of its parts.'

## THE POWER OF REFRAMING

Ever found yourself navigating inner turmoil, when someone asks you, 'How are you?' and you answer, 'Yeah, all right', despite feeling anything but okay inside? As neurodivergents, many of us were given the first-class seat in rumination and intrusive thoughts, not to mention the fact that our past traumatic experiences also have a way of distorting our view of ourselves and how we see the world. But when you find that the stories you've been telling yourself are keeping you small, perhaps you need to change the quality of these stories? In this way, you can go from a state of learned helplessness to learned hopefulness.

Martin Seligman, the founding father of the positive psychology movement, was a self-proclaimed pessimist turned optimist. Seligman initially conducted research on learned helplessness, which focused on how we can learn to feel helpless and powerless in the face of challenging situations. When Seligman presented his research, he was heckled by another academic, who said that there are people in the world, who no matter what life threw at them, would refuse to feel helpless.

Over time, Seligman transitioned his focus from the idea of helplessness to one of hopefulness and identified two key concepts that distinguish individuals who flourish from those who do not:

1. **Learned optimism:** Seligman's research on learned optimism revealed that individuals who cultivate a positive and optimistic outlook are better equipped to navigate life's challenges and achieve greater psychological wellbeing. By changing their explanatory style from pessimistic to optimistic, individuals can learn to approach setbacks with resilience and adaptability. In other words, how we look at negative events in a more positive light and cultivate a sense of hope and agency makes all the difference to our happiness and wellbeing.

2. **Explanatory style/attribution theory:** Seligman's attribution theory focuses on how individuals attribute causes to events in their lives and the impact of these attributions on their emotions and behaviours. By analysing their explanatory style – whether they attribute events to internal or external factors, stable or unstable causes – individuals can gain insight into their thought patterns and develop a more constructive and adaptive way of interpreting experiences. Those with an optimistic explanatory style tend to be happier and more resilient in facing adversity compared to those with a pessimistic explanatory style.

In his 2004 Ted talk, Seligman remarked, 'The skills to heal are not the same as the skills to build a happy life.'[6] He and others realized that the field of psychology helps miserable people recover so that they can live in the day to day. However, to live a happy and meaningful life, we need more than the skills to relieve our misery. We need the skills to create positive emotions, to positively engage with our strengths and apply them to our love, life, family and work, and to devote time to a purpose that is greater than you.

I didn't realize until I wrote this book that the process of learning all about my neurodivergence and how it manifested into mistakes and successes has helped me realize that I have created a sense of peace in the present. Knowing that I was able to learn from my past experiences to improve the way I show up has made me even more hopeful for the future.

Similarly, I hope that a positive reframe of your neurodiverse experiences will condition your body and mind to be optimistic about how things will improve – even when they may not seem so in the present – and to remain hopeful for what is to come. You've spent long enough in the underworld. While this doesn't mean that life will always be easy from here on, you can certainly do yourself a favour and build resilience by choosing to claim your light over darkness. As coach and bestselling author Tony Robbins is fond of saying, 'Where focus goes, energy flows.'

## How to Reframe

On a practical level, reframing your experiences can entail looking at what your challenges might have been in the past and what protected you then. You can then use some of those strategies again now and in the future, whenever the need arises. The table below shows some examples.

| LIFE STAGE | WIDELY REPORTED CHALLENGING FACTORS | LESS PUBLICIZED PROTECTIVE FACTORS THAT BUILD RESILIENCE |
|---|---|---|
| Childhood | • Adverse childhood experiences (ACEs) – abuse or neglect<br>• Post-traumatic stress disorder (PTSD)<br>• Chaotic family home<br>• Challenges with educational attainment<br>• School dropout<br>• Physical, mental and emotional health issues<br>• Behavioural and conduct challenges<br>• Being bullied by siblings, peers or teachers<br>• Hormonal changes during puberty | • Healthy eating<br>• Ways to channel energy (sports, nature, parks)<br>• Parents who get on with each other and nurture you<br>• Nurturing special interests<br>• Presence of charismatic adults, teachers or mentors who nurture your abilities<br>• Positive roles you played in school and community<br>• Positivity sought from books or friends |

*(Continued)*

| LIFE STAGE | WIDELY REPORTED CHALLENGING FACTORS | LESS PUBLICIZED PROTECTIVE FACTORS THAT BUILD RESILIENCE |
|---|---|---|
| | | • Living in a sunny country where naps are normalized and interdependence between family and communities are encouraged |
| Adolescence to Young Adulthood | • Physical, mental and emotional health issues<br>• Conduct disorder<br>• School dropout<br>• Learning disability<br>• Being bullied by peers<br>• Anxiety, depression, eating disorder, body dysmorphia<br>• Self-medicating with alcohol, drugs, sex, partying<br>• Teenage pregnancy<br>• University dropout | • Healthy eating and lifestyle<br>• Abstaining from neurotransmitter-altering substances<br>• Discovering your strengths, talents and skills<br>• Presence of charismatic adults, teachers or mentors who believe in you<br>• Parents who get on with each other and nurture you<br>• Support network of friends, partner and family<br>• Time to explore who you are and what you like<br>• Nurturing special interests |

| LIFE STAGE | WIDELY REPORTED CHALLENGING FACTORS | LESS PUBLICIZED PROTECTIVE FACTORS THAT BUILD RESILIENCE |
|---|---|---|
| | | • Reward of strengths and talent (intelligence, creativity or science and technology skills) in cultures that value academic attainment |
| Adulthood | • Challenges with learning life skills for independent living<br>• Transition into the world of work<br>• Physical, mental, emotional and social challenges<br>• Self-medicating<br>• Emotional distress during transitions<br>• Friendship and relationship fall out<br>• Work dissatisfaction | • Healthy eating and lifestyle<br>• Exploring your interests, talents and skills to find your place in the world of work<br>• Supportive friendships and relationships<br>• Being around positive people with growth-mindset<br>• Spending time on special interests |
| Pregnancy and Childbirth | • Birth trauma<br>• Anxiety about navigating this life stage due to hormonal changes | • The process of matresence or patresence where our brain and body change in preparation for this new phase of life |

*(Continued)*

| LIFE STAGE | WIDELY REPORTED CHALLENGING FACTORS | LESS PUBLICIZED PROTECTIVE FACTORS THAT BUILD RESILIENCE |
|---|---|---|
| | • Postnatal depression and anxiety<br>• Breastfeeding challenges<br>• Lowered confidence in our ability to be a good parent<br>• Overwhelm | • Love and bonding hormones from nurturing your baby<br>• Being able to bring a new life into the world<br>• Supportive partner, family and friends<br>• Living in a sunny country where naps are normalized and interdependence between family and communities are encouraged |
| Menopause | • Hormonal imbalances<br>• Heightened ADHD or autism symptoms<br>• Mood disorders<br>• Borderline personality disorder (BPD), depression, anxiety | • Healthy eating and lifestyle<br>• Adequate hormonal support<br>• Neuroendocrine remodelling, where hormonal and brain changes can lead to a deeper, more mature understanding of others' emotions and perspectives, known as Theory of Mind |

| LIFE STAGE | WIDELY REPORTED CHALLENGING FACTORS | LESS PUBLICIZED PROTECTIVE FACTORS THAT BUILD RESILIENCE |
|---|---|---|
| | | • A supportive partner, family, friends and healthy intimacy<br>• Rite of passage to maturity<br>• Being confident about ourselves and our choices without worrying about what others think<br>• Living in a sunny country where naps are normalized and interdependence between family and communities are encouraged |

The point is, whether your neurodivergence manifests as a strength or disability depends on your experience, which is a combination of your strengths, needs, what particular challenges you faced in certain circumstances, how you look after yourself and the presence of support around you.

## THE VITAL 'A-LIST' TO HELP YOU MOVE FORWARD

As we approach the end of our exploration of the ADHD iceberg together, I would like to share what I call the 8As with you, to help you embrace your new understanding of yourself and navigate the journey ahead.

### 1. Awareness

It all begins with being empowered with the knowledge of how your neurodivergence presents in the unique reality of your individual circumstances and life stage. It is vital to learn from those who share parallel experience with you, having lived in similar cultures, class, race and life stages. Given the high rates for co-occurring forms of neurodivergence, such as ADHD and autism, you will come to see that even if being an ADHDer is an identity you readily resonate with, you will be different to others who share the label. Understanding your specific needs and the preferences of your neurotype will help you to self-advocate in relation to medication, therapy or lifestyle management advice.

### 2. Assurance

I get why you might doubt yourself. After all, your self-esteem has likely taken quite a hit over the years while you've been busy trying to get your brain to do what is required to live in this world. To counter this self-doubt, search through your history and identify key moments in your life when your unique interest (or perhaps obsession) made you good at something, and channel that self-belief and confidence in your ability into your journey from hereon. If you don't currently have faith in yourself, I would borrow this from someone who has your best interests at heart, someone who sees the good and the potential in you, and gives you the assurance you need to take the first step out of your comfort zone. One day, you will embody this belief beyond words.

### 3. Authenticity

To be yourself with integrity and possess the courage to stand alone is a freeing process. You'll always be enough when you come from an authentic place. Being authentic can protect you from feeling rejected or ostracized by people who aren't aligned with your values and morals. However, it's not a linear process, as when you start being true to yourself, this may lead to separation from those closest to you. Even when you know you've valid reasons to travel down your new path, there may be times when you feel the people you love don't want to go on that journey with you. This may frustrate your desire to belong and there may come a time when you doubt if you should be doing this at all. This is where some soul-searching is called for, to go inward and explore the vision you have for your life and the relationships you want to have, your vocation and social circle; it's well worth basing all of this in what you value most. You will find that being true to yourself will help you to develop healthy communication skills when navigating your relationships at work, home and in social groups, and if you join a community of like-minded people. When you are authentic and feel accepted for who you are, it feels like being given the permission to thrive – to be you on purpose.

### 4. Acceptance

There comes a point after you've learned all about yourself that you can begin the process of radical self-acceptance, embracing your unique strengths and needs. You need to reframe your neurodivergence through the lens of self-love, non-judgement and compassion, and realize that some of the traits people say are 'bad' also have a beautiful side to them. For example, your heightened sensitivity also means you're caring and won't give up on others, while your hyperactivity also means an abundance of energy that can light up the entire world when channelled into the right areas. But this isn't a one-and-done job; it's about choosing to accept, love and forgive yourself anew every day. You may also begin to crave acceptance by others and begin to unmask in your own ways, overcoming shame and doubt, honouring your history, making amends and moving forward to become who you were always meant to be.

## 5. Alchemy

This is where your story transforms – where the pain, confusion, shame and rejection are not erased, but transmuted. You start turning your wounds into wisdom, and your survival strategies into sovereign choices.

Through reclaiming a personal narrative that makes meaning of your experiences, reframing your story in a way that honours your growth, wisdom and resilience, and embodied co-regulation practices, you begin to create meaning out of mess, and find power in places you once felt powerless.

This is the part of the journey where you integrate your past – not to stay stuck in it, but to give it purpose. You become the author of your own story, not just the subject of someone else's misunderstanding. Alchemy isn't an ending, it's a continuous practice and a way of living.

## 6. Agency

This is about reclaiming your voice, needs and rhythm. Autonomy is about having the freedom to choose your path – but agency is what gives you the power and tools to actually walk it. For neurodivergents, especially those with a persistent drive for autonomy (often labelled as PDA), the stress of external demands can hijack the nervous systems and lead to serious mental health consequences. In fact, research has shown that 82 per cent of adult autistic PDAers experience severe anxiety, and 84 per cent have contemplated suicide.[7] These statistics aren't about weakness; they reflect how deeply we need choice, safety, and full authority over our own lives. Agency begins by reclaiming our internal authority. That means identifying what matters most to us (values mapping), noticing how our energy and decision-making are affected by things like hormones or sensory overload (hormone-neurotype syncing), using ADHD-friendly tools to support executive functioning and not shaming ourselves for struggling. Claiming agency also means setting boundaries that protect our rhythm and peace. It's saying, 'This is how I move through the world, and I'm allowed to honour that.' We may not always be able to control systemic barriers like class, race, gendered expectations or care work, but we *can* lean into the strengths our neurotype offers – creativity, adaptability, sensitivity and fierce integrity. It's not about being perfect, but an ongoing, courageous practice of aligning with our truth. It's how we break free from generational conditioning and finally start living on purpose – in our own way, on our own terms.

**7. Aliveness**

The need to feel alive. Our neurodivergence leads us to need a deeper reason for our being. This quality isn't imaginary; the terms that can follow many of us through our lives include 'low-frustration tolerance', 'hungry brain', 'sensation-seeking', or 'special interests' – meaning that many neurodivergents continually seek the next big thing that can keep us sufficiently engaged and stimulated. Half of adults with ADHD have spent years relying on substances to cope with seeking that aliveness, even when we know that our self-destructive traits aren't conducive to our quality of life.[8] Heck, evolutionary research even shows us that these 'ADHD-risk alleles' are being phased out of society gradually.[9] Moving forward, finding health means to cater to our need to feel alive, one of our deepest needs. You can perhaps experiment with developing a growth mindset by setting goals for yourself, spending time on your special interests, in play, movement or in exciting intimacy with a regular partner in ways that involve both risk and security, or channelling your energy into a cause or purpose that lights you up.

**8. Affiliation**

Ultimately, we need to realize that while we have differences that set us apart from those who don't share our brain differences, there are inherent similarities between neurodivergents and neurotypicals – we are human beings with the desire for connection, with goals and aspirations, with a capacity for learning, empathy and compassion. Let's recognize and celebrate these similarities, even if we all take different routes to get there. After all, with so much heterogeneity in the neurodiverse population, the lines that separate our differences are going to become increasingly blurred. No one is untouched by life; we have all been through some form of trauma or another. By focusing on what unites us as humans rather than what sets us apart, we can harness our strengths for collaboration within every sphere we live to create a harmonious and supportive environment for everyone, regardless of brain differences. Our world needs all types of minds to work in synergy and interdependence.

## Cultivating a Growth Mindset

Getting an ADHD diagnosis is the start of coming home to yourself. Equipped with your new self-awareness, you get to choose how to live in ways that will bring you joy, alignment, energy, meaning and contentment, rather than self-sabotage and chaos. Take a moment now to consider the following prompts:

1. What lights you up – the stuff that makes you lose track of time or feel fully alive, fully *you*?
2. How could you channel your energy into something that fills your cup instead of draining it?
3. What activities get you into a flow state?
4. How can you bring more of these into your life?
5. What would feel good to work towards this year?
6. What's one tiny step you could take today to start moving?

When considering these questions, there's no pressure or 'shoulds'. Just gentle curiosity and self-trust. Because this new chapter is yours – and it gets to feel good.

I hope this wraps up what feels like a trip into the depths of our collective soul to assist you in doing your own excavation into the hidden world below the tip of your neurodivergence label, so you can emerge ready to take on whatever life throws your way with excitement, joy and authenticity.

# Conclusion: The Journey Ahead

Writing this book and exploring the layers of the ADHD iceberg has felt like unearthing the hidden truths buried beneath the surface of our shared experience with ADHD, with the aim of fostering a deeper understanding of what we're capable of in both our darkness and light.

From our genes to our stories growing up alongside our parents who may or may not have faced similar challenges, in a culture that fed us with what to internalize as the norm, we've often had to find our way very quickly. Despite the vast heterogeneity in our presentations, we share some similarities across different cultures, ethnicity and geographical locations. Some neurodivergent traits are undeniably biologically linked, like the fact that we may experience rejection sensitivity dysphoria (RSD), challenges with working memory, a lack (or not) of resilience to stress, substance use, and a certain way of responding to medication and the impact of our hormones on our moods. On the other hand, some of our traits are a result of an adaptive response to the life that we've had.

As the neurodiversity movement evolves, I am hoping that the advocacy work encompasses an understanding that being born with neurodivergence isn't dissimilar to inheriting traits that influence how our body and brain respond to the world. Like a tendency towards sensitivity, or needing different kinds of nourishment or rest, it's a natural diversity that shapes how we move through life and is very much a part of what it means to be human. Neurodiversity has its place in humanity, and if we can harness the strengths within us and manage our challenges, we have the innate ability to carry humanity into a better world.

Perhaps what had been missing in our lives until now is a contextualized knowledge of what we're dealing with. Even with the awareness that comes with an ADHD or AuDHD diagnosis and the understanding that certain behaviours are inherent to our state of being, many of us still desire to gain better control over things like unexpected outbursts that lead to challenging interactions and a subsequent sense of shame. That's why I was initially motivated to dig deep into the molecular level, some of the known genetic mutations underlying our neurodivergence, and found how they impact the balance of neurotransmitters and metabolites in our bodies, and affect how we show up. And how our life stages can bring about changes that throw our entire systems out of whack.

And it's also why I appreciate the growing field of 'psychiatry with a soul', where we begin to see mental health, neurodivergence and trauma not as a pathology, but as a process. By exploring how both our biology and upbringing influence where we land on the spectrum of complex behaviours – such as how we respond to stress, regulate our emotions, moods and cognitive abilities – we can uncover the underlying causes of observable behaviours and develop customized strategies to navigate our future path more effectively. As Dan Siegel said, 'Awareness is needed for change, and integration is fundamental to achieving wellbeing.'[1] Ultimately, I hope the knowledge you've gleaned in these pages gives you the freedom to choose how you show up, create the life you want for yourself and find the words to advocate for yourself on your way there.

I've come to understand that as we reimagine our lives through the lens of our unique neurodivergent experiences, we must build a raft – one made of self-understanding, compassion and truth. A vessel strong enough to carry us beyond the choppy waters surrounding the ADHD iceberg, and toward the shores of the life we've longed for but never quite knew how to reach. Not just a life of survival – but one rooted in self-trust, belonging and the quiet, radical power of contentment.

# Glossary

**adverse childhood experience (ACE)** – a stressful or traumatic event that occurs during childhood or adolescence.
**affective empathy** – also known as 'emotional empathy'; the ability to understand and share another person's emotions through a sense of connection.
**alexithymia** – an inability to communicate thoughts and feelings.
**amygdala** – regulates emotional salience and social responses; shared across the salience and social brain networks.
**anterior cingulate cortex** – A key part of the salience and executive networks; involved in error detection, impulse management and shifting attention.
**attention deficit hyperactivity disorder (ADHD)** – a neurodevelopmental condition where the brain works differently to the brains of most others. It is typically characterized by persistent patterns of inattention and/or hyperactivity or impulsivity.
**AuDHD** – a distinct neurotype where autistic and ADHD traits co-occur.
**autism spectrum disorder (ASD)** – also known as 'autism'; a neurodevelopmental condition usually characterized by differences in communicating and interacting with others, understanding how they are feeling, and repetitive patterns of behaviour, interests or activities. The term *spectrum* reflects the wide range of experiences and abilities among autistic individuals – from highly verbal to non-speaking, and from needing significant daily support to living independently.
**basal ganglia** – manages movement, habits and reward processing; works with motor and executive networks.
**bipolar** – a mental health condition causing extreme changes in mood with periods of mania and periods of depression, lasting days or weeks at a time.
**borderline personality disorder (BPD)** – a condition of mood and personal interaction traditionally characterized by emotional instability, disturbed patterns of thinking or perception, impulsive behaviour and intense relationships with other. It is a condition rooted in deep emotional sensitivity, often stemming from intense relational experiences and a profound need for connection. People with BPD tends to feel emotions more deeply and for longer than others, and may struggle with regulating these powerful emotional waves.

**cerebellum** – supports balance, coordination and fine motor control, as well as timing and motor learning; part of the motor and sensory integration systems.

**corpus callosum** – enables communication between the left and right hemispheres; supports integration across all brain networks.

**dyslexia** – a common learning difference causing specific challenges with certain skills used for learning, such as reading and writing.

**dyslexithymia** – a tendency to use the wrong words for thoughts and feelings, leading to difficulties with treatment and understanding.

**dyspraxia** – also known as 'developmental coordination disorder'; a common disorder that affects movement and coordination.

**fusiform gyrus** – supports facial recognition and interpretation of facial expressions; part of the social brain network.

**generalized anxiety disorder (GAD)** – a common mental health condition characterized by feelings of anxiety about lots of different things.

**major depressive disorder (MDD)** – a mood disorder causing persistently low or depressed mood or a decreased interest in pleasurable activities.

**neurotype** – the way in which a person's brain processes sensory stimuli and learns, affecting how they perceive the world and communicate.

**obsessive compulsive disorder (OCD)** – a mental health condition where a person has obsessive thoughts and performs compulsive behaviours.

**orbitofrontal cortex** – contributes to decision-making, emotional regulation and interpreting social behaviour; part of the social brain network.

**personality disorder** – a person with a personality disorder thinks, feels, behaves or relates to others differently from the average person. There are several different types.

**post-traumatic stress disorder (PTSD)** – a mental health condition triggered by very stressful, frightening or distressing events, usually characterized by nightmares and flashbacks, insomnia, irritability and guilt.

**prefrontal cortex** – handles planning, attention, impulse control and decision-making; central to the executive network.

**premenstrual dysphoric disorder (PMDD)** – a more extreme form of premenstrual syndrome, the symptoms experienced by many neurodivergent women during the lead up to their period. PMDD symptoms include headaches and joint pain, insomnia, anxiety and depression.

**rejection sensitivity dysphoria (RSD)** – extreme emotional sensitivity to perceived rejection or criticism.

**reticular activating system** – maintains alertness, attention and sensory responsiveness; part of the arousal and salience networks.

**superior temporal sulcus** – processes social cues like gaze direction, body movement, and vocal tone; part of the social brain network.

**Tourette syndrome (TS)** – a neurodevelopmental condition causing someone to make involuntary, sudden, repetitive sounds or movements (tics). Tics are usually triggered by stress, excitement or tiredness.

# Source Notes

## INTRODUCTION

1. See my story at www.linkedin.com/posts/samanthahiew_audhd-neurodivergence-autisticwomen-activity-7314889692607307777-G0I2?utm_source=share&utm_medium=member_desktop&rcm=ACo AAAQghJQBEOu98rmM0BcLY2Sxggi3Kfgzafw
2. 'Eight-year ADHD Backlog at NHS Clinics Revealed' (July 2024), available at https://www.bbc.co.uk/news/articles/c720r1pxrx5o?

## STEP 1: UNDERSTAND IT'S NOT YOUR FAULT

1. 'Neurodiversity and Increasing Risk Of Tribunals' (December 2023), available at https://www.business-reporter.co.uk/human-resources/neurodiversity-and-increasing-risk-of-tribunals (accessed September 2024)
2. Spencer T, Biederman J and Mick E, 'Attention-deficit/hyperactivity disorder: Diagnosis, lifespan, comorbidities, and neurobiology', *Journal of Pediatric Psychology*, 2007, 32(6), 631–42
3. Hinshaw SP, 'Preadolescent girls with attention-deficit/hyperactivity disorder: I. Background characteristics, comorbidity, cognitive and social functioning, and parenting practices', *Journal of Consulting and Clinical Psychology*, 2002, 70(5), 1086–98
4. 'Hundreds of Thousands More Women Tested for ADHD Last Year' (January 2022), available at https://www.independent.co.uk/news/uk/home-news/adhd-women-gender-differences-b1993364.html (accessed September 2024)
5. Russell G et al, 'Time trends in autism diagnosis over 20 years: A UK population-based cohort study', *Journal of Child Psychology and Psychiatry*, 2022, 63(6), 674–682

6. McCrossin R, 'Finding the proportion of females with autistic spectrum disorder who develop anorexia nervosa, the true prevalence of female ASD and its clinical significance', *Children*, 2023, 10, 272
7. *International Statistical Classification of Diseases and Related Health Problems* (ICD) (2025), available at https://www.who.int/standards/classifications/classification-of-diseases (accessed April 2024)
8. 'The People Behind DSM-5-TR' (2022), available at https://www.psychiatry.org/getmedia/5635958b-ee71-4352-b02a-fb24ecab86c6/APA-DSM5TR-ThePeopleBehindDSM.pdf (accessed April 2024)
9. Ecks S, 'The strange absence of things in the "culture" of the DSM-V', *Canadian Medical Association Journal*, 2015, 188(2), 142–3
10. Hens K and Van Goidsenhoven L, 'Developmental diversity: Putting the development back into research about developmental conditions', *Frontiers in Psychiatry*, 2023, 13, 986732
11. 'Meeting the Needs of Neurodiverse Students' (2023), available at https://www.unitegroup.com/neurodivergent-students-report (accessed April 2024)
12. Mueller AK et al, 'Stigma in attention deficit hyperactivity disorder', *Attention Deficit Hyperactivity Disorder*, 2012, 4(3), 101–14
13. 'Number of ADHD Patients Rising, Especially Among Women' (2023), available at https://www.epicresearch.org/articles/number-of-adhd-patients-rising-especially-among-women (accessed April 2024)
14. Attoe DE and Climie EA, 'Miss. Diagnosis: A Systematic Review of ADHD in Adult Women', *Journal of Attention Disorders*, 2023, 27(7), 645–57
15. Magdi HM et al, 'Attention-deficit/hyperactivity disorder and post-traumatic stress disorder adult comorbidity: A systematic review', *Systematic Reviews,* 2025, 14 (41)
16. 'Research Domain Criteria', available at https://www.nimh.nih.gov/research/research-funded-by-nimh/rdoc
17. Dodson W, 'Emotional Regulation and Rejection Sensitivity', (October 2026), available at https://d393uh8gb46l22.cloudfront.net/wp-content/uploads/2016/10/ATTN_10_16_EmotionalRegulation.pdf (NB: The claim that children with ADHD receive approximately 20,000 more negative messages by age 12 is widely cited in ADHD literature and advocacy. This estimate is often attributed to psychiatrist Dr. William W. Dodson, who has discussed the cumulative impact of negative feedback on children with ADHD. However, the exact methodology behind this figure isn't detailed in peer-reviewed studies, it serves to highlight the frequent criticism and correction these children may experience.)

## STEP 2: EXPECT TO DISCOVER CO-OCCURRING CONDITIONS

1. Ursino M et al, 'Bottom-up vs. top-down connectivity imbalance in individuals with high-autistic traits: An electroencephalographic study', *Frontiers in Systems Neuroscience*, 2022, 16, 932128
2. 'A New Picture Of Autism in Girls is Emerging, Says Gina Rippon', available at https://www.newscientist.com/video/ 2475916-a-new-picture-of-autism-in-girls-is-emerging-says-gina-rippon
3. Panagiotidi M, Overton PG and Stafford T, 'Co-occurrence of ASD and ADHD traits in an adult population', *Journal of Attention Disorders*, 2019, 23(12), 1407–15
4. 'Decoding the Overlap Between Autism and ADHD' (2018), available at https://www.thetransmitter.org/spectrum/ decoding-overlap-autism-adhd/?fspec=1
5. Rommelse NN et al, 'Shared heritability of attention-deficit/hyperactivity disorder and autism spectrum disorder', *European Child and Adolescent Psychiatry*, 2010, 19(3), 281–95
6. Dougherty CC et al, 'A comparison of structural brain imaging findings in autism spectrum disorder and attention-deficit hyperactivity disorder', *Neuropsychology Review*, 2016, 26(1), 25–43
7. Koirala, S., Grimsrud, G., Mooney, M. A., Larsen, B., Feczko, E., Elison, J. T., Nelson, S. M., Nigg, J. T., Tervo-Clemmens, B., & Fair, D. A. (2024). *Neurobiology of attention-deficit hyperactivity disorder: Historical challenges and emerging frontiers.* Nature Reviews Neuroscience. https:// url.de.m.mimecastprotect.com/s/3dGTCnRLmvFm9026fZs2iJ6Jak? domain=doi.org
8. Hull, J. V., Dokovna, L. B., Jacokes, Z. J., Torgerson, C. M., Irimia, A., & Van Horn, J. D. (2017). Resting-State Functional Connectivity in Autism Spectrum Disorders: A Review. *Frontiers in Psychiatry*, 7, 205. https://url. de.m.mimecastprotect.com/s/IFIZCoZMnwTv2NRKuOtNip5JzM?dom ain=doi.org
9. 'The AuDHD Expert: 3 Alarming Risks of Undiagnosed Female AuDHD', available at https://www.youtube.com/ watch?v=QfOSKl2iLTQ
10. Watanabe D and Watanabe T, 'Distinct frontoparietal brain dynamics underlying the co-occurrence of autism and ADHD', *eNeuro*, 2023, 10(7), ENEURO.0146-23.2023
11. Young S et al, 'Guidance for identification and treatment of individuals with attention deficit/hyperactivity disorder and autism spectrum disorder based upon expert consensus', *BMC Medicine*, 2020, 18(1), 146

12. Festinger L, 'A theory of social comparison processes', *Human Relations*, 1954, 7(2), 117–40
13. 'Can CBT be Helpful for Autistic Adults? Part 1' (December 2023), available at https://attwoodandgarnettevents.com/can-cbt-be-helpful-for-autistic-adults-part-1/ (accessed June 2024)
14. Rydén E et al, 'Mapping phenotypic and aetiological associations between ADHD and physical conditions in adulthood in Sweden: A genetically informed register study', *The Lancet Psychiatry*, 2021, 8(9), 774–783
15. Oluwabusi OO, Parke S and Ambrosini PJ, 'Tourette syndrome associated with attention deficit hyperactivity disorder: The impact of tics and psychopharmacological treatment options', *World Journal of Clinical Pediatrics*, 2016, 5(1), 128–35
16. Cravedi E et al, 'Tourette syndrome and other neurodevelopmental disorders: A comprehensive review', *Child and Adolescent Psychiatry and Mental Health*, 2017, 11, 59
17. 'The Dyslexia–ADHD Overlap: Why Evaluators Confuse the Conditions' (2025), available at https://www.additudemag.com/dyslexia-evaluation-adhd-comorbidity-overlap/ (accessed June 2025)
18. 'Autism and Dyslexia: Is There a Connection?' (2023), available at https://www.abtaba.com/blog/autism-and-dyslexia
19. 'The Overlap Between Dyspraxia, Dyslexia and ADHD', available at https://psychiatry-uk.com/the-overlap-between-dyspraxia-dyslexia-and-adhd/ (accessed June 2025)
20. 'Dyspraxia and Autism: Shared Symptoms' (2023), available at https://www.bridgecareaba.com/blog/dyspraxia-and-autism (accessed June 2025)
21. 'ADHD and Dyscalculia' (2005), available at https://www.academia.edu/111744001/ADHD_and_Dyscalculia (accessed June 2025)
22. Soares N and Patel DR, 'Dyscalculia', *International Journal of Child and Adolescent Health*, 2015, 8(1), 15–26
23. Garcia-Argibay M et al, 'Attention-deficit/hyperactivity disorder and major depressive disorder: Evidence from multiple genetically informed designs', *Biological Psychiatry*, 2024, 9(5), 444–52
24. 'Major Depressive Disorder in Autism Spectrum Disorder: A Double Whammy' (2021), available at https://www.psychiatrist.com/pcc/major-depressive-disorder-autism-spectrum-disorder/ (accessed June 2025)
25. Hudson CC, Hall L and Harkness KL, 'Prevalence of depressive disorders in individuals with autism spectrum disorder: A meta-analysis', *Journal of Abnormal Child Psychology*, 2019, 47, 165–75
26. Quenneville A F et al, 'Anxiety disorders in adult ADHD: A frequent comorbidity and a risk factor for externalizing problems', *Psychiatry Research*, 2022, 310, 114423

27. Hudson CC, Hall L and Harkness KL, 'Prevalence of depressive disorders in individuals with autism spectrum disorder: A meta-analysis', *Journal of Abnormal Child Psychology*, 2019, 47, 165–75
28. Pehlivanidis A, Papanikolaou K, Mantas V et al. 'Lifetime co-occurring psychiatric disorders in newly diagnosed adults with attention deficit hyperactivity disorder (ADHD) or/and autism spectrum disorder (ASD)', *BMC Psychiatry* 20, 423 (2020), available at https://doi.org/10.1186/s12888-020-02828-1
29. Spera V et al, 'Substance use disorder in adult-attention deficit hyperactive disorder patients: Patterns of use and related clinical feature', *International Journal of Environmental Research and Public Health*, 2020, 17(10), 3509
30. Ahlberg R et al, 'Prevalence of sleep disorder diagnoses and sleep medication prescriptions in individuals with ADHD across the lifespan: A Swedish nationwide register-based study', *BMJ Mental Health*, 2023, 26, 1–8
31. Huisman-van Dijk HM et al, 'The relationship between tics, OC, ADHD and autism symptoms: A cross-disorder symptom analysis in Gilles de la Tourette syndrome patients and family-members', *Psychiatry Research*, 2016, 237, 138–46
32. For more on ADHD mental health and physical health conditions, visit www.additudemag.com
33. For more on ASD mental and physical health conditions, visit: www.autism.org.uk
34. Quoted in 'Modern Concepts of ADHD – Peter Hill', available at https://youtu.be/hGlTEMyEmcw?si=DPlXU8gOqu2lGALz (accessed April 2024)
35. Meyer HC and Leeh FS, 'Translating developmental neuroscience to understand risk for psychiatric disorders', *American Psychiatric Association*, 2019, 176(3), 171–252
36. 'Funding Agency Seeks to Dismantle Diagnostic Barriers' (December 2017), available at https://www.thetransmitter.org/spectrum/funding-agency-seeks-to-dismantle-diagnostic-barriers/?fspec=1 (accessed May 2024)
37. Katzman MA et al, 'Adult ADHD and comorbid disorders: Clinical implications of a dimensional approach', *BMC Psychiatry*, 2017, 17(1), 302
38. Duffy KA et al, 'Increased integration between default mode and task-relevant networks in children with ADHD is associated with impaired response control', *Developmental Cognitive Neuroscience*, 2021, 51, 100988
39. 'ADHD is a Whole-Life Experience. The DSM Needs to Reflect That' (May 2024), available at https://www.additudemag.com/emotional-dysregulation-dsm-5-adhd-women (accessed May 2024)
40. 'Modern Concepts of ADHD', available at https://www.youtube.com/watch?v=hGlTEMyEmcw (accessed June 2025)

41. For more on this, see Seligman M, *What You Can Change and What You Can't: The Complete Guide to Successful Self-Improvement* (2007) Vintage, London
42. Maté G, *The Myth of Normal: Trauma, Illness and Healing in a Toxic Culture* (2022), Penguin, New York

## STEP 3: UNDERSTAND YOUR NATURE

1. Thapar A, 'Discoveries on the genetics of ADHD in the 21st century: New findings and their implications', *American Journal of Psychiatry*, 2018, 175(10), 943–950
2. Yadav SK et al, 'Genetic variations influence brain changes in patients with attention-deficit hyperactivity disorder', *Translational Psychiatry*, 2021, 11, 349
3. Palmer CM, *Brain Energy: A Revolutionary Breakthrough in Understanding Mental Health – And Improving Treatment for Anxiety, Depression, OCD, PTSD, and More* (2022) Simon and Schuster, New York
4. Meyer HC et al, 'Translating developmental neuroscience to understand risk for psychiatric disorders', *American Journal of Psychiatry*, 2019, 176(3), 179–185
5. Tottenham N and Sheridan MA, 'A review of adversity, the amygdala, and the hippocampus: A consideration of developmental timing', *Frontiers in Human Neuroscience*, 2010, 3, 68
6. Xie C, Xiang S, Shen C et al, 'A shared neural basis underlying psychiatric comorbidity', *Nature Medicine*, 2023, 29, 1027–1037
7. 'Long-term ADHD Treatment Increases Brain Dopamine Transporter Levels, May Affect Drug Efficacy' (May 2013), available at https://medicalxpress.com/news/2013-05-long-term-adhd-treatment-brain-dopamine.html (accessed May 2024)

## STEP 4: TRACE YOUR BEGINNINGS

1. Long M et al, 'New gene evolution: Little did we know', *Annual Review of Genetics*, 2013, 47, 307–33
2. Hartmann T, *ADHD: A Hunter in a Farmer's World* (2019), Healing Arts Press, Vermont
3. Esteller-Cucala P et al, 'Genomic analysis of the natural history of attention-deficit/hyperactivity disorder using Neanderthal and ancient Homo sapiens samples', *Scientific Reports*, 2020, 10(1), 6522

4. Barack D et al, 'Attention deficits linked with proclivity to explore while foraging', *Proceedings of the Royal Society B: Biological Sciences*, 2024, 291(1998), 20222584
5. Esteller-Cucala P et al, 'Genomic analysis of the natural history of attention-deficit/hyperactivity disorder using Neanderthal and ancient Homo sapiens samples', *Scientific Reports*, 2020, 10(1), 6522
6. 'Women with ADHD: No More Suffering in Silence' (March 2025), available at https://www.additudemag.com/gender-differences-in-adhd-women-vs-men/ (accessed May 2024)
7. James O, *They F\*\*\* You Up: How to Survive Family Life* (2005), Hachette, New York
8. Storebrø OJ et al, 'Association between insecure attachment and ADHD: Environmental mediating factors', *Journal of Attention Disorders*, 2013, 20(2) 187–196
9. Eyuboglu M and Eyuboglu D, 'Emotional regulation and attachment style in previously untreated adolescents with attention deficit and hyperactivity disorder', *Dusunen Adam Journal of Psychiatry and Neurological Sciences*, 2020, 33, 228–36
10. Crandall A A et al, 'ACEs and counter-ACEs: How positive and negative childhood experiences influence adult health', *Child Abuse & Neglect*, 2019; 96, 104089
11. Bethell C et al, 'Adverse childhood experiences, resilience and mindfulness-based approaches: Common denominator issues for children with emotional, mental, or behavioral problems', *Child and Adolescent Psychiatric Clinics of North America*, 2016, 25(2), 139–56
12. Charabin E, ' "I'm doing okay": Strengths and resilience of children with and without ADHD', *Journal of Attention Disorders*, 2023, 27(9), 1009–19
13. Charabin E, ' "I'm doing okay": Strengths and resilience of children with and without ADHD', *Journal of Attention Disorders*, 2023, 27(9), 1009–19
14. Menakem R, *My Grandmother's Hands: Racialized Trauma and the Pathway to Mending Our Hearts and Bodies* (2021), Penguin, New York
15. Mosconi L et al, 'Menopause impacts human brain structure, connectivity, energy metabolism, and amyloid-beta deposition', *Scientific Reports*, 2021, 11, 10867
16. Gold EB et al, 'Factors related to age at natural menopause: Longitudinal analyses from SWAN', *American Journal of Epidemiology*, 2013, 178(1), 70–83
17. Gottardello D and Steffan B, 'Fundamental intersectionality of menopause and neurodivergence experiences at work', *Maturitas*, 2024, 189, 108107
18. Eng AG et al, 'Attention-deficit/hyperactivity disorder and the menstrual cycle: Theory and evidence', *Hormones and Behavior*, 2024, 158, 105466

19. De Jong M et al, 'Female-specific pharmacotherapy in ADHD: Premenstrual adjustment of psychostimulant dosage', *Frontiers in Psychiatry*, 2023, 14, 1306194
20. Eng AG et al, 'Attention-deficit/hyperactivity disorder and the menstrual cycle: Theory and evidence', *Hormones and Behavior*, 2024, 158, 105466
21. 'Women with ADHD: No More Suffering in Silence' (March 2025), available at https://www.additudemag.com/gender-differences-in-adhd-women-vs-men/ (accessed May 2024)
22. 'Inclusion and Advocacy for Women with ADHD: Addressing Inequities and Challenging Diagnostic Bias on International Women's Day' (2023), available at https://www.acamh.org/blog/inclusion-and-advocacy-for-women-with-adhd-addressing-inequities-and-challenging-diagnostic-bias-on-international-womens-day/ (accessed May 2024)
23. Nøvik TS, ADORE Study Group et al, 'Influence of gender on attention-deficit/hyperactivity disorder in Europe – ADORE', *European Child and Adolescent Psychiatry*, 2006, 15(Suppl 1), i15–i24
24. 'Doctor Gabor Maté: I Regret My Interview with Prince Harry! The Shocking Link Between Kindness & Illness!' (2023), available at https://podcasts.apple.com/us/podcast/doctor-gabor-mate-i-regret-my-interview-with-prince/id1291423644?i=1000631046969 (accessed May 2024)
25. Peng P-H et al, ' Attention-deficit/hyperactivity disorder, its pharmacotherapy, and adrenal gland dysfunction: A nationwide population-based study in Taiwan', *International Journal of Environmental Research and Public Health*, 2020, 17(10), 3709
26. Lembke A, *Dopamine Nation: Finding Balance in the Age of Indulgence* (2021), Penguin, New York
27. Ram Dass quotes available at https://www.ramdass.org/ram-dass-quotes/

## STEP 5: IDENTIFY YOUR EMOTIONAL NEEDS

1. Long Z et al, 'Alteration of functional connectivity in autism spectrum disorder: Effect of age and anatomical distance', *Scientific Reports*, 2016, 6, 26527
2. Watanabe D and Watanabe T, 'Distinct frontoparietal brain dynamics underlying the co-occurrence of autism and ADHD', *eNeuro*, 2023, 10(7), ENEURO.0146–23.2023
3. Ochoa J, *Focused Forward: Navigating the Storms of Adult ADHD* (2016), Empowering Minds Press
4. Spencer AE et al, 'Examining the association between posttraumatic stress disorder and attention-deficit/hyperactivity disorder: A systematic review and meta-analysis', *Journal of Clinical Psychiatry*, 2016, 77(1), 72–83

5. Rumball F, Happé F and Grey N, 'Experience of trauma and PTSD symptoms in autistic adults: Risk of PTSD development following DSM-5 and non-DSM-5 traumatic life events', *Autism Research*, 2020,13(12), 2122–32
6. Barbier A, Chen J H and Huizinga J D, 'Autism spectrum disorder in children is not associated with abnormal autonomic nervous system function: Hypothesis and theory', *Frontiers in Psychiatry*, 2022,13, 830234
7. Spencer A E et al, 'Abnormal fear circuitry in Attention Deficit Hyperactivity Disorder: A controlled magnetic resonance imaging study', *Neuroimaging*, 2017, 262, 55–62
8. Panksepp J, 'Affective neuroscience of the emotional BrainMind: Evolutionary perspectives and implications for understanding depression', *Dialogues in Clinical Neuroscience*, 2010, 12(4), 533–45
9. Ibid.
10. Van der Kolk B, *The Body Keeps the Score: Brain, Mind, and Body in the Healing of Trauma* (2014) Penguin, New York
11. Maté G, *The Myth of Normal: Trauma, Illness and Healing in a Toxic Culture* (2022), Penguin, New York
12. See their website at https://energyaccounting.com/about/
13. Maté G, *The Myth of Normal: Trauma, Illness and Healing in a Toxic Culture* (2022), Penguin, New York

## STEP 6: EXPECT YOUR RELATIONSHIPS TO CHANGE AND ADAPT

1. 'How to Foster Lasting, Healthy Relationships in Your Life, According to Famed Therapist Esther Perel' (February 2024), available at https://fortune.com/well/article/esther-perel-lasting-health-relationships/ (accessed July 2024)
2. Quoted at www.relationallifefoundation.org/sliding-scale-relational-life-therapy.html?utm_source=chatgpt.com (accessed July 2024)
3. Duarte M et al, 'Adult ADHD and pathological narcissism: A retrospective-analysis', *Journal of Psychiatric Research*, 2024, 174, 245–253
4. For further information, visit https://www.rcpsych.ac.uk/mental-health/mental-illnesses-and-mental-health-problems/personality-disorder?utm_source=chatgpt.com
5. Allely C S, Woodhouse E and Mukherjee R A, 'Autism spectrum disorder and personality disorders: How do clinicians carry out a differential diagnosis?', *Autism*, 2023, 27(6), 1847–50
6. Ibid.
7. Adamis D et al, 'Prevalence of personality disorders in adults with Attention Deficit Hyperactivity Disorder (ADHD)', *Journal of Attention Disorders*, 2023, 27(7), 658–668

8. Palmer C, *Brain Energy: A Revolutionary Breakthrough in Understanding Mental Health* (2023), St Martin's Press, New York
9. Allely CS, Woodhouse E and Mukherjee RA, 'Autism spectrum disorder and personality disorders: How do clinicians carry out a differential diagnosis?', *Autism*, 2023, 27(6), 1847–50
10. Damian RI et al, 'Sixteen going on sixty-six: A longitudinal study of personality stability and change across 50 years', *Journal of Personality and Social Psychology*, 2019, 117(3), 674–95
11. Siegel DJ, *Personality and Wholeness in Therapy: Integrating Nine Patterns of Developmental Pathways in Clinical Practice* (2021), WW Norton, New York
12. Mulder R and Tyrer P, 'Borderline personality disorder: A spurious condition unsupported by science that should be abandoned', *Journal of the Royal Society of Medicine*, 2023, 116(4), 148–50
13. Ibid.
14. Lewis CR et al, 'Pilot study suggests DNA methylation of the glucocorticoid receptor gene (NR3C1) is associated with MDMA-assisted therapy treatment response for severe PTSD', *Frontiers in Psychiatry*, 2023, 14, 959590
15. Konowałek Ł and Wolańczyk T, 'Attachment and executive functions in ADHD symptomatology: Independent inputs or an interaction?', *Brain Science*, 2020, 10(11), 765
16. The Attachment Project, Mead, 2023, available at www.attachmentproject.com (more specifically, The Attachment Project stated that disorganized attachment is more likely in children with ASD)
17. Erkoreka L et al, 'Genetics of adult attachment: An updated review of the literature', *World Journal of Psychiatry*, 2021, 11(9), 530–42
18. Cavicchioli M et al, 'The role of attachment styles in attention-deficit hyperactivity disorder: A meta-analytic review from the perspective of a transactional development model', *European Journal of Developmental Psychology*, 2022, 20(3), 436–64
19. Coughlan B et al, 'Differentiating "attachment difficulties" from autism spectrum disorders and attention deficit hyperactivity disorder: Qualitative interviews with experienced health care professionals', *Frontiers in Psychology*, 2022, 12, 780128
20. Antunes GF et al, 'Dopamine modulates individual differences in avoidance behavior: A pharmacological, immunohistochemical, neurochemical, and volumetric investigation', *Neurobiology of Stress*, 2020, 12, 100219
21. Downey G and Feldman SI, 'Implications of rejection sensitivity for intimate relationships', *Journal of Personality and Social Psychology*, 1996, 70(6), 1327–43

22. Cacioppo S et al, 'A quantitative meta-analysis of functional imaging studies of social rejection', *Scientific Reports*, 2013, 3, 2027

## STEP 7: NAVIGATE YOUR NEURODIVERSITY AT WORK

1. '45% of the C-Suite Identify as Neurodivergent – Here's Why Businesses Should Care' (January 2024), available at https://www.unleash.ai/learning-and-development/45-of-the-c-suite-identify-as-neurodivergent-heres-why-businesses-should-care/ (accessed September 2024)
2. 'Bosses Urged to Help Neurodiverse Workers Thrive'(March 2024), available at https://iosh.com/news-and-opinion/bosses-urged-to-help-neurodiverse-workers-thrive (accessed September 2024)
3. 'Workplace Neurodiversity Claims Spur Companies to Seek Legal Help' (March 2024), available at https://www.ft.com/content/29728b03-ffac-49c0-a98b-f1f372328175 (accessed September 2024)
4. McDowall A, Doyle N and Kiseleva M, *Neurodiversity at Work: Demand, Supply and a Gap Analysis* (2023), Birkbeck, University of London, London
5. For information and inspiration, visit https://cityandguildsfoundation.org/what-we-offer/campaigning/neurodiversity-index/ and https://www.autistica.org.uk/get-involved/employers/ndei#:~:text=The%20Neurodiversity%20Employers%20Index%20(the,a%20leader%20in%20workplace%20neuroinclusion
6. 'How Employee Resource Groups Can Unleash The Powers Of Neurodiversity' (July 2024), available at https://www.peoplemanagement.co.uk/article/1882640/employee-resource-groups-unleash-powers-neurodiversity (accessed September 2024)

## STEP 8: FIND YOUR COMMUNITY

1. Van der Kolk B, *The Body Keeps the Score: Brain, Mind, and Body in the Healing of Trauma* (2014) Penguin, New York
2. 'Mental Health, Human Rights and Legislation: Guidance and Practice' (October 2023), available at https://www.who.int/publications/i/item/9789240080737
3. See https://www.gov.uk/access-to-work

## STEP 9: EMERGE AS YOUR TRUE SELF

1. 'Have We Been Thinking about ADHD All Wrong?'(April 2025), available at https://www.nytimes.com/2025/04/13/magazine/adhd-medication-treatment-research.html
2. See https://ifs-institute.com/resources/articles/internal-family-systems-model-outline
3. Siegel DJ, *IntraConnected* (2022), W W Norton, New York
4. Available at https://drdansiegel.com/wheel-of-awareness/
5. 'Mental Health, Human Rights and Legislation: Guidance and Practice' (October 2023), available at https://www.who.int/publications/i/item/9789240080737
6. 'The New Era of Positive Psychology' (February 2004), available at https://www.ted.com/talks/martin_seligman_the_new_era_of_positive_psychology?language=en
7. 'PDA: Lives Worth Living – A Report About the Experiences of PDA Adults' (May 2023), available at https://www.pdasociety.org.uk/research-professional-practice/pda-lives-worth-living/
8. 'Half of Adults with ADHD Have Had a Substance Use Disorder' (August 2021), available at https://www.eurekalert.org/news-releases/924775
9. Esteller-Cucala P et al, 'Genomic analysis of the natural history of attention-deficit/hyperactivity disorder using Neanderthal and ancient Homo sapiens samples', *Scientific Reports*, 2020, 10, 8622

## CONCLUSION

1. See https://www.eliseloehnen.com/episodes/dan-siegel

## Acknowledgements

**Writing this book saved me during some of the most difficult times in my life.** When everything I once knew disintegrated, knowing I could return to this project felt like an anchor on my journey.

It carried me through countless transitions – growing my social impact company ADHD Girls, navigating a divorce, learning to co-parent, enduring heartbreaks, nurturing new and genuine friendships, moving twice and shaping each space into something that felt like mine, and walking myself back to self-love. It's been a journey of discovering what it means to feel truly alive, to be present in my body, and to belong to myself again.

When I began writing this book, I felt an enormous sense of responsibility to get it right. That feeling intensified when I started researching the ADHD experience and realized how little I actually knew when I first began speaking about it. The truth is, our neurodivergent experiences carry profound depth – shaped by unique contexts, intersections, and the environments we move through.

I learned this the hard way: through suffering, and then healing. I was so trapped in my head – so disconnected from my body – that it took extreme emotional pain to pull me back into myself. That's when I realized: you can't think your way through this journey. You have to live it. Feel it. Make space for all of your emotions and the community of inner parts that will sometimes work in harmony, and sometimes feel at war. And then learn to strike a balance between noticing your internal world and remembering that there is life out there too.

I had no idea how profoundly my life would change with that ADHD diagnosis in 2021. And with that, I must thank the people and events that rocked my world and gifted me the wisdom to grow in ways I never imagined possible.

**To my children, Raphie and Leo** — You are my greatest loves and my greatest teachers. Thank you for showing me how to show up, for reminding me to soften, and for enabling me to create the space within to be both a mother and a woman.

**To every romantic relationship that shaped a season of my life** – thank you. Each of you brought something real: passion, pain, curiosity, chaos, beauty. You mirrored back parts of me I hadn't yet learned to hold – especially the hidden layers of my autistic ADHD experience. When the noise faded and I was left to navigate the silence alone, that's where my deepest learning lived.

Through the emotional turmoil, I finally cracked open and began to feel in my body what had eluded me for decades.

Over time, I came to see it not as failure, but as transformation. Each relationship became a mirror, helping me track the patterns that won't shift – until we start living in full alignment with our neurotype, nervous system and truth.

They taught me what I truly value: not just safety. Not just aliveness. But love that feels like oxygen – not suppression. A space where the voice that had been buried could finally rise. And from this place, I now create spaces where others can exhale, unmask and come home to themselves.

**To my therapist, Nancy Wilson** — You were the true spark behind my life shake-up nearly three years ago. You've helped me reconstruct a stronger identity, clarified my values, and reminded me that I do have a strong sense of self when nothing seems certain. Every time I think I'm ready to leave therapy, something happens. The work is never done – and that's okay.

**To my 'crystal ball', Lyn Birkbeck** — Thank you for your honesty. I needed to hear it, even if it took you saying it eight times before I believed it. You introduced me to the (frankly whacky) idea of 'finding stability by getting the hang of change', which describes the AuDHD experience immensely. You've helped me settle into being the 'one of a kind' human you said I am, on this planet.

**To my editor, Lou** — An intersectional feminist and all-round kick-ass woman. You believed in this book before I even knew what was going into these pages. Thank you for translating my tornado of thoughts into a structure my AuDHD brain could follow – you made the book feel possible. Thanks as well to the wordsmiths Sue Belfrage and Joanna Smith, and the wonderful Octopus team: Rimsha Falak, Mel Four, Sarah Parry, Ailie Springall and Charlotte Sanders.

**To the clinical psychologists, Heidi and Clodagh** — Thank you for *not* giving me an autism diagnosis the first three times – it made me dig deeper and gave me the motivation to truly understand the science underlying the AuDHD experience. So when you finally gave me the diagnosis at the fourth appointment, it completed the story for me as an intersectional AuDHD woman. I've since developed the first intersectional and scientific training programme to support professionals like you – people with the power to transform how unseen and unrecognized AuDHDers are supported.

**To my biology teacher, Mrs Fun** — Thank you for sparking my love of biology. It still brings me enormous comfort when I try to make sense of life and people – because just like science, everything in life is a process.

**To Professor Chong-Lek Koh** — You made me fall in love with genetics – a subject many find mind-numbing, but you made it come alive. Imagine being able to read the very code of life.

**To my friends Suresh, Leanne and Camilla** — Your friendship helped me break free from the old conditioning, and it mirrored back the part of me that feels deeply and still reaches for the sky. You helped me release years of suppression and healed me more deeply than any modern medicine ever could.

**To my family in Malaysia – Mummy, Daddy, Jarod, Hanny, Brennan and Nicole** — Thank you for being my safe space. No matter how far I roam, I know I can always come home to you and rest my head. I love you all.

**To the neurodiverse community and women everywhere** — Through you, I've found my place in the collective. I've held space and had it held for me. We've learned, cried, healed together, and washed away old wounds in each other's presence. Through this journey, I've found my purpose: to work towards a new society that recognizes ADHD, autism and neurodivergence not as deficits, but as natural and brilliant variations of the human genome. Not less. Just different. Just extraordinary.

# Index

Glossary entries have suffix 'g'

## A

acetylcholine 123, 124
addiction 134–5, 183
ADHD 6–7, 10, 20–6, 269–71, 303g; in adults 57–8, 68; and ASD 3, 42–9, 55–6, 60–7; and the brain 46–7, 57, 63, 85–9, 147–8; causes 80–3, 195; holistic view of 252–5, 271–87; and personality disorders 189–94; personality traits 192–4, 226–9, 253–4, 301; symptoms 15–16, 77, 270–1; treatment 29–31, 270; underrepresented groups 7–8, 19, 21, 25–6, 119, 132, 263
adolescents 86–9, 290–1
adrenals/adrenaline 90–1
adverse childhood experiences (ACEs) 87, 92, 115–17, 156–7, 303g
affective empathy 61, 182, 303g
agency, claiming 296–7
alexithymia 10, 61, 95, 170, 182, 303g
amygdala 46–7, 85–6, 90, 147, 148, 303g
anterior cingulate cortex 47, 303g

anxiety 53, 63, 86, 304g
ASD. *see* autism spectrum disorder (ASD)
assurance 294
attachment styles 115–16, 183, 200–5
attention span 66
attribution theory 288
AuDHD 44–9, 56, 60–7, 187, 271–5; and the brain 148–50; personality traits 226–9, 253–4; and relationships 197–8
auditory processing disorder (APD) 56
authenticity 10, 37, 140, 144–5, 172–3, 215–18, 295; impact of diagnosis 183–6; vs belonging 161, 268; vs interdependence 286
autism spectrum disorder (ASD) 20, 153–4, 213–14, 303g; and ADHD 3, 42–9, 55–6, 60–7; and the brain 46, 148; causes of 195; male-centric models 43–4; and personality disorders 194; personality traits 42, 50, 226–9; and relationships 196–7
autonomic nervous system (ANS) 90, 149, 150–1, 213; window of tolerance 154, 159, 164–5, 278–82

## B

basal ganglia 47, 148, 303g
bipolar 49, 64, 96, 303g
blood sugar levels 99, 100, 102, 103
borderline personality disorder (BPD) 190, 198–9, 303g
bottom-up thinking 41, 65, 148
the brain 46–7, 50–1, 57, 147, 154–6; and ADHD 46–7, 57, 63, 85–9, 147–8; and AuDHD 45, 47–8, 63, 65–6, 148–50; and autism 46, 148
brain energy theory 84

## C

CBT (Cognitive Behavioural Therapy) 30–1
cerebellum 46, 47, 147, 148, 304g
challenges 114–15; ACEs 87, 92, 115–17, 156–7, 303g; cultural differences 117–20; gender 120–9; internalizing negativity 33–5, 116, 118–19, 128–9; race, ethnicity and class 129–32; self-medicating 103, 132–6; social expectations 126–9, 273
change 103–4, 160, 264–8, 273; and ADHD 64, 103–4; and AuDHD 62
children 19, 43–4, 55–7, 172; brain development 85–9; importance of support 87–8, 116–17
class 132
co-occurring conditions 9, 26–8, 51–8; mental 41–9, 53–4; physical 52, 54–5, 81–3, 89–90
co-regulation 60, 151
communication skills 231–3, 243–5, 259–61, 285
comorbidities 48–9. *see also* co-occurring conditions
compassion-focused therapy 168–72
control 62, 63, 67, 73–5
coping strategies 58, 72, 132–6, 138, 271–94
corpus callosum 46, 47, 304g
culture: and ADHD 117–20; differences in 21, 22–6, 119, 129, 132

## D

decision paralysis 95, 162
demand avoidance 63, 66, 67, 203
depression 53, 213–14
diagnosis 3–4, 7–9, 16–24, 31, 32, 34. *see also* labelling; ableist assessment 50–1; cultural differences 22–6; impact of 13–16, 28–9, 32–3, 183–6, 249–50; increases in 7–8, 20
diet 99–101, 113, 126
dissociation 88, 138, 150, 155
dopamine 78, 83, 86, 135–6; and medication 94, 187; and oestrogen 122–3, 124, 188; and stress response 91, 93
DSM-5 and DSM-5-TR (*Diagnostic and Statistical Manual of Mental Disorders*) 20–4, 45, 68, 193, 269
dyscalculia 53
dyslexia 53, 56, 304g
dyslexithymia 10, 61, 95, 170, 304g
dyspraxia 53, 56, 85, 304g

### E

emotional dysregulation 68, 86–7, 116, 156–60, 182, 200–1, 281
emotional needs 143; and the brain 147–50; compassion-focused therapy 168–72; polyvagal theory 150–2; recognizing your reality 162–4; risks of suppressing 161–2; sensory overload 166–8; survival response 152–6; unmet 145–6
emotional systems 157–60, 196
emotions 61, 154, 159, 164–5, 213, 275–82, 284–5
empaths 200–1
empathy 61, 182, 191–2
energy 81–4, 104
energy accounting 166–8
environment 88, 273–4
Equality Act 2010: 239–42, 243
ethnicity 129–32
executive function 57, 88, 101, 123–4, 182
exercise 102, 103, 126

### F

fear 154–6
fight or flight response 90–1
frontal cortex 87–8
frontal lobe 50–1, 65, 85, 89
fusiform gyrus 46, 304g

### G

gender and ADHD 120–9
generalized anxiety disorder (GAD) 53, 63, 304g
genetic influences 80–3, 104, 107–11, 139, 274
girls 19, 20, 43–4
glimmers 213
global majority groups 26
grieving process 29
gut health 99, 101

### H

healing 37, 38, 179–81
health professionals 25, 269–70
health reviews 102–3
hippocampus 147, 148
homeostasis 84, 89–90, 98
hormones 83, 103, 122–6, 188, 267
hypothalamus 90–1

### I

ICD-11 (*International Classification of Diseases*) 20–4, 105
identity, finding 32–3, 58–67, 275–8
impact of diagnosis 13–16, 28–9; facing shame 33–5; finding identity 32–3; grief cycle model 184–6; on relationships 183–6; stigma and negative messages 34–5
impulsivity 183
inflammation 103
insulin resistance 103
interdependence 286
Internal Family Systems (IFS) model 275–8
intersectionality 118–19, 240–1, 245–6

## J

journaling 73, 101, 104, 141

## L

labelling 16–17, 31; and co-occurring conditions 26–8; and cultural differences 24–6; definitions of ADHD 20–4; and negative language 48–9; and personality disorders 190, 198
language, negative 48–9
lifestyle 98–103
limbic system 85, 147, 149
limerence 183
low frustration tolerance 183

## M

major depressive disorder (MDD) 49, 53, 304g
masking 24–6, 43–4, 62, 129–32
medial prefrontal cortex 46
medication 30, 78–9, 93–7, 187–9, 213, 270
meditation 281–2
men 3, 43–4, 120, 261–2
menopause 122, 267, 292–3
menstrual cycle 79, 123–4, 125
mental health conditions 9, 20–4, 26–8, 48–9. *see also* individual conditions; causes 195–200; holistic approach 252–5, 271–87
metabolic pathways 81–3
metabolites 82, 84
metacognition 50–1
mind deficit theory 182

mindset 111–12, 298
mitochondria 83
monotropism 183, 221
motor skills 85
MTHFR gene 82–3

## N

narcissists 189–92, 200–1
nature vs nurture 10, 274
negative messages, reframing 34–5
nervous system 90–1, 147–8; and ADHD 91–3, 154–6; regulating 102, 279
neurobiology 45–8, 81–3
neuroception 151
neurodivergents 3–4, 114–15, 265–6, 283–4. *see also* individual conditions
neuroplasticity 87, 114, 197–9
neurotransmitters: and gene variants 82; increased levels 30, 59, 60, 78, 91; and medication 93, 97, 187
neurotype 93, 304g
norepinephrine 78, 86, 93, 94, 187–8
nurture. *see* environment
nutrition 98, 99–101, 113

## O

obsessive compulsive disorder (OCD) 53, 63, 304g
oestrogen 122–3, 126, 188
optimism 287
orbitofrontal cortex 46, 304g
oxidative stress 103

## P

parasympathetic nervous system (PNS) 90, 149, 150
parenting 137, 159, 201–2
past, reframing 37, 289–93
patterns of developmental pathways (PDP) 195–6
PCOS (polycystic ovary syndrome) 83
PDA (persistent drive for autonomy) 30–1, 67, 296
personality disorders 189–92, 304g; and ADHD personality traits 192–4; emotional pathways 197–9; neurodevelopmental conditions 195–200
physical health conditions 52, 54–5, 81–3, 89–90
play, power of 172–6
PMDD (premenstrual dysphoric disorder) 83, 123, 304g
polyvagal theory 150–2
prefrontal cortex 46, 147, 304g; development delay 57, 63, 86–8, 148, 156
psychiatrists, role of 21–2
PTSD 153, 304g

## R

race 129–32
radical acceptance 38
recognition responsive euphoria (RRE) 234
reframing 34–5, 37, 226–9, 259, 263–4, 287–93, 296
rejection sensitivity dysphoria (RSD) 10, 16, 182, 212–14, 234, 304g
relationships 10, 61, 62–3, 67, 102, 138, 172–3, 177–8, 285; attachment styles 201–5; and authenticity 215–18; communication 231–3, 243–5, 259–61; conflict 200–1; difficulties 182–3; evaluating 207–11; familial 209–10; and healing 179–81; and medication 187–9; and mental health conditions 195–200; neurodiverse 181–6; and personality disorders 189–94; reflecting on 205–7; rejection sensitivity dysphoria 212–14; romantic 178–9, 208–9; social 210; workplace 188–9; with yourself 207–8
resilience 116–17, 234, 287–93
reticular activating system 47, 85, 148, 304g

## S

self-acceptance 295–6
self-awareness 35–9, 50–1, 68–73, 101, 215–18
self-compassion 38, 277–8
self-esteem 33, 277–8, 294
self-forgiveness 38, 277–8
self-knowledge 50, 68–75, 111–12, 136–42, 275–82
self-medicating 103, 132–6

sensitivity. *see* rejection sensitivity
dysphoria; sensory
overload
sensory overload 62, 166–8, 183,
280
sensory sensitivity 42, 56, 91, 96
serotonin 83, 97, 123, 124
shame 33–5, 226–9
sleep 53, 102
social anxiety 61
Social Comparison Theory 50
social environment 11, 21, 119, 126–9,
263–4, 273
social interaction and AuDHD 60
societal expectations 126–9, 273
stereotypical traits 24–6
stigma 18–19, 20, 28–9, 33–5, 49, 118,
259, 263–4
stress 78–80, 90, 103, 131; and
ADHD 91–3; and autism 153–4;
and lifestyle changes 98–101,
103–4; and lifestyle insights 101–3;
medication review 93–7
substance misuse 103
substance use disorder (SUD) 53
superior temporal sulcus 46,
304g
supplements 93, 97, 98
support networks 249–50; benefits of
11, 251–3, 254–6, 272–3; finding
256–8
survival response 87–8, 152–6
sympathetic nervous system (SNS)
90, 93, 149, 150

T
Theory of Mind deficit 50,
182
therapy 30, 37, 168–72, 188
Tourette Syndrome 53, 304g
trauma 27–8, 180, 199, 273;
intergenerational 111, 119–20, 139;
PTSD 153, 304g; reframing
287–93; stress response 93, 153,
160
treatment options 29–31, 270

V
vagus nerve 92, 150–2
ventral striatum 86

W
window of tolerance 154, 159, 164–5,
278–82
women 2–4, 68, 120–9; attitudes
towards 126–9; hormonal changes
83, 93, 99, 122–6, 188, 267;
personality disorders 190;
relationships 197–8
workplace 11, 65, 188–9, 219–22,
226–9, 230; challenges & barriers
224–6, 263–4; communication in
231–3, 243–5; employee resource
groups 243, 244, 245–7; inclusion
241–2; performance feedback
233–6; supportive strategies
234–42
World Health Organization (WHO)
252–5, 271–87

# RAISING READERS
### Books Build Bright Futures

Dear Reader,

We'd love your attention for one more page to tell you about the crisis in children's reading, and what we can all do.

Studies have shown that reading for fun is the single biggest predictor of a child's future life chances – more than family circumstance, parents' educational background or income. It improves academic results, mental health, wealth, communication skills, ambition and happiness.[1]

The number of children reading for fun is in rapid decline. Young people have a lot of competition for their time. In 2024, 1 in 10 children and young people in the UK aged 5 to 18 did not own a single book at home.[2]

Hachette works extensively with schools, libraries and literacy charities, but here are some ways we can all raise more readers:

- Reading to children for just 10 minutes a day makes a difference
- Don't give up if children aren't regular readers – there will be books for them!
- Visit bookshops and libraries to get recommendations
- Encourage them to listen to audiobooks
- Support school libraries
- Give books as gifts

There's a lot more information about how to encourage children to read on our website: www.RaisingReaders.co.uk

Thank you for reading.

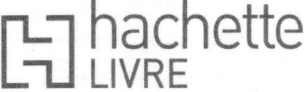

---

[1] OECD, '21st-Century Readers: Developing Literacy Skills in a Digital World', 2021, https://www.oecd.org/en/publications/21st-century-readers_a83d84cb-en.html

[2] National Literacy Trust, 'Book Ownership in 2024', November 2024. https://literacytrust.org.uk/research-services/research-reports/book-ownership-in-2024